HOLD
— THE —
PHONE

AVONSIDE
PRESS

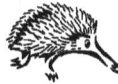

HOLD
— THE —
PHONE

THE DEFINITIVE GUIDE TO
HOW TO PROTECT YOUR HEALTH
FROM PHONES AND WIRELESS

ALISON WILSON

AVONSIDE
PRESS

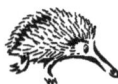

First published in 2013 by Avonside Press

Copyright © 2013 by Alison Wilson

Although the author and publisher have made every effort to ensure that the information in this book was correct at press time, the author and publisher do not assume and hereby disclaim any liability to any party for any loss, damage, or disruption caused by errors or omissions, whether such errors of omissions result from negligence, accident or any other cause.

This book is not intended as a substitute for the medical advice of physicians. The reader should consult a physician in matters relating to his/her health and particularly with respect to any symptoms that may require diagnosis or medical attention.

ISBN: 978-0-9922865-6-9

Illustration on page 141 reproduced with the kind permission of Om P Gandhi, University of Utah, USA.

Avonside Press Pty Ltd
PO Box 356, North Manly, NSW 2100
Australia

To the boys
Tim, Oliver, and Toby

*The future depends entirely
on what each of us does every day.*

Gloria Steinem

Contents

FOREWORD

It was December 1992, some twenty years ago, when the first public questions about a possible link between mobile phones and brain cancer were raised. On the United States syndicated television show *Larry King Live*, neurologist Dr David Perlmutter stunned the world with an X-ray showing a brain tumor in his patient, Susan Reynard, juxtaposed to the area where she held her mobile phone close to her head.

In those days, mobile phones were the size of bricks, very expensive, and used primarily by early technology adopters and those with above-average financial means. Her husband, David, who was in the telecommunications business and wanted to provide a convenience for her during a difficult pregnancy, gave Susan Reynard the phone. The tumor was fatal and the family brought suit against the phone industry for negligence.

The Reynard family claimed that the industry knew of the dangers from wireless radiation and did not warn consumers. Above the mobile phone industry's adamant claims that there was no danger - the industry's mantra was "thousands of studies prove cell phones are safe" - telecommunications stocks tumbled, congressional hearings were held, and a decades-long search for scientific answers ensued.

My job was to run what remains the world's largest research effort into mobile phone dangers: seven years, fifty-six separate studies, US government oversight, and $28.5 million in funding from the mobile phone industry itself.

At the conclusion of that program in June 1999, we recommended to the government in the US and the global telecommunications industry that, given surprising evidence that mobile phones caused genetic damage in human blood, disruptions of brain physiology, and increases in the risk of rare brain tumors, warnings to consumers were warranted.

Those warnings, which would have empowered consumers to make their own informed safety choices while the health risk questions were sorted out with necessary follow-up science, never came.

A decade later, the majority of mobile phone users around the world remain unaware of the inherent dangers they subject themselves and their families to every day through their mobile phone use - dangers elucidated by serious and well-conducted scientific studies.

Today, my personal library contains more than seventeen thousand scientific papers relevant to the question of mobile phone health effects. It is now evident that even in the early 1990s, there was science - though not all in the public domain - that was indicative of impending health risks from mobile phone-like radiation.

The science today is quite clear. There are real dangers. The good news is that these dangers are manageable in most cases - wired-headsets remain the best protection tool.

Wireless technology is one of the most rapidly evolving and changing technologies in history. The cell phones of the 80s and 90s were very different from the smartphones of today. And, that means that over time the exposures to people have changed, the biological effects have changed, and the scientific tools to assess what those changes in exposure and effect mean to public health are necessarily changing as well.

This presents a significant challenge to government, industry and the scientific community who are doing their best to figure it all out. It is important to keep that in mind when reading this book. Pay close attention to the dates affixed to specific quotes cited. What we know today is much more complete than what we knew in 2001 or 2007 or 2010. And, we will know more next year and the year after.

It is this dynamic that underscores an important message:

While the science is being sorted, precaution makes sense.

The axiom "knowledge is power" has particular relevance here. And this is precisely why this knowledge-conveyance book by Alison Wilson should be read by, and remain on the bookshelf of, every parent, spouse, and friend of every person who uses mobile communication devices.

As a concerned and energetic parent, spouse, and friend, Alison has done what governments, scientists, and industry have so far failed to do: empower consumers to make their own informed safety choices about wireless communication devices.

She has done a rigorous job sorting through the volumes of science, the quotes of countless experts, and the sometimes-diversionary paths offered by vested industry, scientific, and government groups. The result is an easy-to-understand fact book that allows you, the reader, to draw your own conclusions about what this science means, how best to manage the risks, and thereby take steps to protect those closest to you.

Sometimes it is simply best to take matters into your own hands. Alison Wilson has done just that, and this book allows you to do the same. Well done, Alison . . .

G L Carlo
August 2013

INTRODUCTION

*"There is nothing to fear
except the persistent refusal to find out the truth."*

Dorothy Thompson

The Basics
How this book works

This book is half of a companion set of books: *'Hold The Phone'* and *'Hold The Phone: Here's Why'*. Read together they will:

➢   allow you to make an informed choice about your future

➢   give you everything you need to know to help yourself

Both books are based on the words and work of credible, experienced, and independent experts in the fields of science, public health, and mobile telecommunications technology.

Why's it a good idea to have both books? Because together they will give you the complete picture - everything you need to know about *what* to do, and *why*.

This book - Hold The Phone - will give you quick and easy tips on *how* to protect your health. This is the 'good news' book. Packed full of simplesolutions, it will show you: *who* the experts are,

➢   the message they have been trying to get to you,

➢   the steps they're advising you to take, and, most importantly,

➢   how just a few little changes can make a big difference

The second book - Hold The Phone: Here's Why - will let you in on *why* that's a good idea. This is the 'reference' book. It will lay the facts and the evidence out for you so that you can clearly see:

➢   what the concerns are about using mobile phones (and cordless phones and wireless appliances too),

➢   how phone use can affect your health, and what the real-life symptoms look like,

➢   the basics of how this technology works,

➢   what the science has found,

- what the experts are saying,

- and the many public warnings that have already been issued around the globe.

The reference and resources section at the back of both books will let you know:

- the reliable sources that you can trust for accurate information,

- the references and websites that will help you to do your own research,

- where to go if you want to learn more about radiation and health issues, and

- who to call if you want someone to assess your exposure to radiation at home or in the office.

Clear and simple: Both books have been clearly and simply laid out so that you can cut to the chase, get to the facts, and find out exactly what to do: *quickly and easily.*

"Our lives begin to end the day we become silent about things that matter."

Martin Luther King Jr

The Bottom Line
Why Read a Book Like This?

We've all heard the health concerns raised about mobile phones.

Reading this book will show you the best ways of preventing them from compromising *your* health.

Does that mean that you'll be asked to stop using your phones? No, because realistically, that's probably not going to happen. Instead, by finding out how to use them more *wisely*, you'll learn how to minimize their effect on you.

A friend told me that when the 'Pill' first became available in the '70s, she went to ask her doctor for a script. She'd already set her course of action into place; all she wanted was help with protection. His answer, because she was young and unmarried, was that "the best contraceptive is the word *'No!'*". His refusal to accept the reality of the situation, or offer her practical advice, left her exposed and vulnerable.

The parallel is obvious. We have to accept what is. There is little point in attempting to tell anyone, especially teenagers, "just say no to mobile phones". It's not going to happen. What is likely to happen is that they'll quietly slope off and do it anyway - without protection. We need to show them what to do to protect themselves.

What the world does not need now is another stern, fear-based book that waves its finger at you and tells you what's terrible about the way in which you live. Chances are you probably have enough on your plate already.

What *is* needed now is pragmatism and acceptance, followed up with practical advice. A solution-focussed approach, with good health as its main goal.

This book is not attempting to convince anyone of anything. Rather, it's there for those who are already aware of concerns about phones and wireless - *and just want to know what to do about it*.

Following the tips given in this book may well help if you feel any of the following:

➢ difficulty in focussing, concentrating, and remembering

➢ anxiety, irritability, or nervousness

➢ restlessness and the inability to relax

➢ palpitations or arrhythmia

➢ headaches

➢ dizziness and nausea

➢ sick and tired of feeling sick and tired

➢ at the end of your tether because you can't get a good night's sleep

The effects can be cumulative, so every time you follow these tips it will make a difference. Each and every little step truly does help.

Even if you're lucky enough not to feel any of these symptoms yet, following these simple steps will help to *prevent* you from experiencing them in the months and years to come.

This book will present material that enables you to make an educated decision about your own future. Not everyone's decision will be the same, but it will allow you to find out the truth about the issues and make an informed choice. *Your* choice.

"There is inadequate warning and notice to the public about possible risks from wireless technologies in the marketplace, which is resulting in adoption and use of technologies that may have adverse health consequences which are still unknown to the public.

There is no 'informed consent'."

The BioInitiative Report *(2007) (1)*

---

1.   Pass it on and help spread the word

The 'Hold The Phone' books are primarily intended as a reference and a resource to help you help yourself.

They are also a resource that you can give to partners, friends, colleagues, and teenagers - *especially* those that are sceptical. It will take the pressure off both of you.

Because they can hear the words directly from the mouths of the many experts, they'll quickly be able to understand the issues and see the validity of the material for themselves.

Because of the *volume* of research and reference materials presented here, they'll see this is fact, and not just opinion. They'll *get* it, without you having to expend energy trying to convince them.

By passing this vital information on to anyone you care about, you'll be creating your own ripple in the pond, and helping to spread the word further around the world.

"You may never know what results come from your action.
But if you do nothing, there will be no results."

Gandhi

WHY *WRITE* A BOOK LIKE THIS?

I wrote this book because phones and wireless are changing our lives in ways that very few people yet realise.

From the research that's been carried out so far, it seems possible that - because it has the potential to affect so many billions of people so quickly - mobile telecommunications is the biggest health issue in the world today.

I've sat by the sidelines waiting for someone to write this book - a simple guidebook on what to do to protect your health. And so far, no one has. There are solid books out there that focus on what's *wrong* with phones and wireless, but the information can be overwhelming and frightening - and it can be difficult to easily extract the remedies.

Everyone is so busy nowadays that they want practical answers - and quick, simple ones at that. That is my intention with this book.

I also believe that people have a right to informed choice, and the ability to safeguard their health. I've been lucky enough to have access to information that most people don't know about. Information that can change health and prolong lives. It felt like something I needed to share.

As with many people who are involved in health and wellbeing, I developed a real interest in health only when mine was threatened. I became ill, and had absolutely no understanding of what had happened, or how I could get better.

I used to have what I thought was a bulletproof constitution. We moved into a brand-new house, and I watched my health disintegrate. As quickly and simply as that. I didn't sleep, constantly felt terrible, and developed allergies until I became intolerant to almost everything. Fast forward a couple of years, and I ended up with chronic fatigue syndrome as well. No energy, a business to run, and two small children is not a good combination.

I didn't know what was wrong with me, and neither did my doctors. I didn't know what to do, nor did they. The only thing I *did* know was that I had no energy. So I decided to find some.

I researched and discovered that there was a whole different perspective on 'health'. Science points to electrical energy as being fundamental to all living matter. Because of that energy is also the basis of *our* health. As an example, if the bio-electrical energy of our body and its communication system is interrupted in any way our natural ability to self-heal can be impaired, often leading to disease.

Because I wanted to understand more about how this affects us, I spent the following years pursuing studies and personal research into the question of energy and its effect on our health. As my level of knowledge improved, so did my health.

Then we moved house, and my young son became very sick. Luckily, by then I knew someone who could help me find out what was wrong. It turned out my son's bed was against the wall next to the electric meter box. He was sleeping in a cloud of electromagnetic radiation. I moved the bed. He got better. Very quickly. The 'cure' was as simple as that.

My son's brush with ill health was relatively short, but I know enough now to understand just how very fortunate we were. Had I not had the vital information about what was interrupting his health, it could have been a very different story - as it is for many.

For me, it was a light bulb moment. I saw in an instant how our *homes* can make us sick. We spend a lot of time there. Despite all the things we *are* doing to stay well, if our home is an unhealthy environment, our immune systems can become overburdened; and many of us end up getting sick. I had to find out more. But where to look?

There's not too much information 'out there' about just how much the buildings in which we live and work affect us. I found one place that resonated. One place that offered information and education on exactly this subject. The Institute of Building Biology and Ecology (IBE). I signed up for the distance education programme, and entered into a whole new world.

Having qualified at their entry level, I was invited to take my studies further and become a Building Biology professional. The next step was to participate in face-to-face week-long seminars: three separate ones, held at different times of the year. The only problem? The IBE was based in the USA. And I wasn't.

Sometimes in life, no matter how much something seems impossible, the pull to do it is so strong that you just have to jump off that cliff. So I signed up for my frequent flyer miles and set off into the very expensive unknown to learn. And learn I did. So much more than I could ever have imagined.

I learnt fact after fact about how toxic influences like the chemicals and electromagnetic radiation in our buildings are stressing us, and stripping so many people of their health. We heard one case study after another of how people had been able to turn their health around simply by changing sometimes very simple things in their homes. (Like moving the bed away from the meter box.)

From that very first day on the Building Biology course with Larry Gust, Spark Burmaster, and Martine Davis, I learnt about all the things that had potentially led to my health imploding. I learnt that - due to all the chemicals present in new building, decorating and furnishing materials, and pest treatments - brand-new houses can be a real threat to our health.

Houses just like the one I'd been living in when I got sick. Combine that with high electromagnetic fields coming from wiring and electrical appliances and the environmental cocktail can be an overwhelming assault on a sensitive immune system.

I took that knowledge, applied the changes suggested to my own home, and watched my health start to move onto a different level again.

Mostly I sat through these lectures feeling as if I were in a parallel universe. If all these facts were *known*, if they were so well recorded that they were actually being *taught*, how come it wasn't general knowledge? Why didn't we all know these simple things as a matter of course? So that *everyone* who had a home knew the things to look out for. So that everyone had the chance to protect or recover their health.

I left the very first seminar series determined to learn as much as possible so that I could help other people understand the extent to which their homes can affect their health - and what they can do about it.

Much has been written about chemicals, and most people have *some* level of understanding that exposure to these toxins can harm their health. But it's a rare individual who knows anything about electromagnetic radiation (EMR).

It felt like I should make that my focus. However, the more I learnt about the effect that EMR has on our health, the more I discovered that there was another issue - an even more widespread health issue. And that is the radiation that's the core of our mobile telecommunications technology. The radiofrequency microwave radiation that's used to operate the mobile phones, cordless phones, and wireless devices that are making our life so convenient has the very real potential to damage our health.

Yet it's very hard to get to the truth of the matter. And it's even harder to find out what to do.

Here was something that was hailed by leading experts in the field as being "the biggest human experiment - ever", and yet no one was really talking openly about it. There were a few weighty and very technical books that had been published, but little that was clear and simple enough to really show those who knew nothing what they could do.

Since graduating from the IBE's professional training as a Building Biology Environmental Consultant (BBEC), and later from the Safe Wireless Initiative of the Science and Public Policy Institute as a Certified Electromagnetic Radiation Safety Advisor (CERSA), I've gone to work.

I've consulted in people's homes, which can be both frustrating and heart-rending. It's impossible not to be touched when you're with someone whose life has been turned upside down because they're not well - especially when you're looking into the eyes of a small child, or consoling a distraught parent.

These aren't case studies or statistics. They are real people who can't make the most of their lives because they simply aren't well enough to do so.

The lives of the parents, friends, and partners who love and care for them are also in turn deeply affected. Everyone's happiness is diminished. As you listen to their stories, you feel your heart melt.

Sometimes it's frustrating, because it's clear that the cause of their ill health has been something very simple. It's just that they haven't known what to do. There is nothing better than being able to pass on information that leads to someone recovering their health. It's beyond deeply fulfilling. Sometimes it seems like a miracle because the 'cure' is so simple and effective that they start feeling better very quickly.

It's not uncommon to suggest a simple change like moving a bed to the other side of a room, or turning off a cordless phone, and then have someone who hasn't been able to sleep for *years* start to sleep that very same night.

I've spent my time trying to get the message and information across as best as I can. As well as consulting, I've held public talks, private talks for professionals, written in magazines, talked on radio, and even appeared on TV - and each time the response has been the same: "Why don't we know about this?" and "Where's the book? You need to write all this down in a book for everyone."

So I did. I took time out and wrote. And then wrote, and wrote even more. I now have the basis of a series of books - all showing people how their homes affect their health - and what they can do about it.

These two 'Hold the Phone' books are the very first because I feel that letting people know - right here, right now - what they can do about mobile phones, cordless phones, and wireless is the absolute, most urgent priority.

My intention with these books? To pass on the favour someone once did me. To give *you* the information that can help you to protect the health of your child, your partner, your parents, your friends, yourself . . . so that you can lead as healthy and happy a life as possible.

And, as you'll see, sometimes the changes needed to facilitate that can be really quick and easy.

As the parent of a young child who was once ill, I'm particularly interested in doing all I can for our children. They are in our care, they rely on us, and they deserve the very best future that we can give them. Hopefully, this will help to make a difference.

We also need to work *together* as communities. Phones and wireless devices all emit a cloud of radiation that can fill the air in neighbourhoods. There are steps we can all take to clean up our own homes, but by talking to neighbours and working together we can make entire communities even safer for everyone.

The information held within these pages does not originate from me. It comes to you from the experts: scientists, public health advocates, electrical engineers, and other specialist professionals.

I'm not an expert, just an informed voice who is acting as the messenger. My job has been firstly to learn and understand, and then to collect, consolidate, simplify and pass on what the experts have been trying to bring to your attention.

These two books may look simple, but that is their deliberate intent. In reality the information here is the distillation of many years of research and study. It's taken that long to accumulate the information and then present it in a way that allows you to get to the priorities without having to wade through acres of stodgy text or technical geek-speak.

It seems as if humanity is at a crossroads at the moment; and the decisions we each make are critical not only to our own health, but also to that of future generations. By making wise choices now, I believe we all still have time to bring about the best future possible.

My hope is that reading these books will open a door for you so that you can move towards a better tomorrow. My hope is that they will empower you with knowledge that you can use to keep yourself healthy.

I wish you all the best in the world with it.

Alison Wilson
August 2013

THE STATUS QUO:
IT IS WHAT IT IS

As with everything in life, there is little point in discussing 'if only'. We just have to deal with what is. The reality that is in front of us right now.

Currently, we have been presented with technology that previous generations could only dream of. And it has to be said that it's not all bad.

Some of the advantages of our new technology are very real, and it's undoubtedly been important to our progression as a society. It's:

> given us freedom: millions are no longer tied to their homes or offices waiting for that very important phone call, and no one needs to know whether you're behind a desk or on the beach.

> changed where we live and work: we now have access to endless information whether we're in a city café or on a country farm.

> allowed us rapid growth: multi-million dollar companies can now be run entirely from a mobile phone and laptop.

> saved us money: releasing us from the burden of costly overheads.

> saved us time: information can be instantly accessed via a few clicks.

> educated us: we have access to an unparalleled amount of information, all of which is increasing exponentially.

> made us more self-reliant: with all this information, we no longer have the need for so many middlemen. From DIY to design, we're able to find out how to go it alone.

> revolutionised social interaction: for youth today, their phone or laptop is the gateway to their peer group. Not to have that access is social suicide

➢   enabled us to keep in contact with each other: despite the arguments on the quality of this contact, and the benefits of instant access 24/7, we're able to communicate real-time with anyone, anywhere. Lost touch with someone decades ago? No problem: in a few seconds, you can track almost anyone down.

However, we also have to remember that the mobile phone industry is a business. They are there to sell phones and keep their shareholders happy. They are there to make money. Individuals or companies who are negligent in doing that face loss of income, loss of employment, and even the prospect of legal action.

Mobile phone companies are not there to look after your health. (Fewer and fewer people seem to be these days.) That is your job.

At the beginning of 2012, it was estimated that there were over six billion mobile phone subscriptions - and climbing. This is not a passing trend.

In terms of health, the best-case scenario is no exposure to radiofrequency/ microwave radiation at all. But we're already way past that. So we need to accept the situation for what it is. The best way forward now is to find out what we need to do to cope with our exposure levels.

As in anything that makes life 'easier', there's often a drawback. By knowing what those drawbacks are, and how to avoid them, you'll be better prepared - and safer.

We each need to learn how to minimise that exposure as best as we can - and that involves taking precautions.

Our mobile telecommunications technology *does* offer us unparalleled convenience. And yes, inviting this technology into our homes and offices *has* changed our lives. Just not necessarily in the way we thought it would.

> *"Most studies, including ours, show we do see something happening in what we call long-term users.*
>
> *As a specialist in public health, I say why shouldn't we take simple measures just to be on the safe side to limit exposure, especially when we are having so many children who are using them?"*
>
> **Siegal Sadetzki** *(2009) (2)*

"We are called to be architects of the future,
not its victims."

Buckminster Fuller

The Takeout
What to take Away from this

Change is the only constant

The science behind wireless technology is a moveable feast: it keeps changing and evolving. We know more today than we did yesterday. And that will be the same tomorrow. And the day after that . . .

What's presented here is not attempting to be a *fait accompli*. It is a report on the most important points that the scientists have found up till now, so that you can see for yourself what's been discovered.

As you read this our knowledge will already have advanced. The dates on the quotes will further highlight the way in which new discoveries are constantly being made.

Because of this, please bear in mind that each of the quotes made by the scientists represents a frozen moment in time. In many cases their knowledge has expanded and matured since the quotes were made – and it will keep on changing. . .

No smoke without fire.

It may be an old warhorse but "there's no smoke without a fire" is very relevant here.

After twenty years of research there is a lot of smoke. It appears that there's a fire in there somewhere. We just don't have all the answers about it yet.

While the scientists attempt to find out where it might be burning, the type of wood that it could contain, the size of the logs, how combustible they are, the factors that might have made it ignite in the first place, what could be keeping it burning, how long fires could be projected to burn for, and which firefighters make up the best team to call in – we need to keep ourselves from choking on the smoke, and possibly getting burnt too.

But, at the end of the day do you really need to know all that before you take evasive action? If there was a wildfire around your corner, would you wait patiently in front of the computer for all those questions to be answered?

Probably not. The solution is the same here. Get out of the environment, and do everything you can to protect yourself while the professionals work on it. They'll get back to you later with the details.

That's the impetus behind the Precautionary Principle – which is the main message to take from this book.

Do everything you can to protect yourself while scientists, governments, and industry work together to sort it all out.

"It is not the strongest of the species that survives,
nor the most intelligent that survives.
It is the one that is the most adaptable to change."

Charles Darwin

THE CAST OF CHARACTERS:

Scientists and Health Experts quoted in this book

The men and women who are issuing the warning

*"In a time of universal deceit,
telling the truth becomes a revolutionary act."*

George Orwell

The Scientists and Health Experts Quoted in this Book

"The ultimate measure of a man is not where he stands in moments of comfort and convenience,
but where he stands at times of challenge and controversy."

Martin Luther King Jr

The information in this book is based on the lifetime's work of highly qualified and experienced professionals.

They come from all walks of life: science, electronics, public health, activism, medicine, alternative health, investigative journalism, building biology, and academia. Some of them have a veritable alphabet of letters after their names; others speak from years of in-field observation and experience.

They all speak from the heart. They are each here because they have a valid and worthwhile contribution to make - and they care.

Whilst coming from many varied and divergent perspectives, they all have three things in common:

1. Whilst professionals in their work life, at home they are just like us: fathers, mothers, siblings, friends, lovers, neighbours, and friends … They are all *people*.

2. They have all found the courage to speak out in the face of the considerable PR spin and marketing coming from the trillion-dollar mobile/wireless industry. Please don't underestimate the bravery of being a lone voice like that: a very small David in the face of an extremely powerful and well-funded Goliath.

3.   They share a heartfelt and compassionate desire to let us know what they have discovered. They are all trying to draw your attention to the potential health issues associated with being exposed to the microwave radiation and radio frequency radiation used in cell phone, cordless phone, and wireless communications technology. Their clarion call? "Use them with extreme caution".

Following are the experts who have been quoted in this book.

In the course of writing this book, I have relied upon information from, and opinions of, many professionals and others who have been at the forefront of addressing the science and public policy aspects of the issue of mobile phone health effects.

I have tried my very best to evaluate their information and opinions from the perspective of their relevant experience, and their specific contributions. I have weighed their opinions based on this information and am providing it here for you, so that you have the opportunity to assess these perspectives for yourself.

Following are the four categories that I have defined and used in preparing this book - and the people who I have assessed to fall within these categories.

1   *The Health Effects Research Scientists*

➢   *Scientists who have conducted their own research studies into RF radiation/cell phones and published their research in peer-reviewed journals*

➢   *Scientists who have reviewed and evaluated other people's research studies into RF radiation/cell phones and published their opinions in peer-reviewed journals*

Alvaro Augusto A de Salles

Professor, Department of Electrical Engineering, Universidade Federal do Rio Grande do Sul (UFRGS), Porto Alegre, Brazil. His special interests include mobile telecommunications and the biological effects of non-ionizing radiation. Member of International Commission for Electromagnetic Safety (ICEMS)

Andrew Goldsworthy

Biologist with special interest in the biological effects of electromagnetic radiation; honorary lecturer in biology, Imperial College London, UK (retired)

Bengt Arnetz

Director, Division of Occupational and Environmental Health, Department of Family Medicine and Public Health Sciences, Wayne State University, Detroit, USA; founder of Center for Environmental Illness and Stress, Academic Hospital, Uppsala, Sweden. His specialty is community-based occupational and environmental health research.

David O Carpenter

Public health physician, professor at the School of Public Health, co-editor of the BioInitiative Report (2007 and 2012), and director of the Institute for Health and the Environment at the University of Albany in New York, USA. In the 1980s, he was executive secretary of the New York State Powerlines Project, the first to replicate the Wertheimer-Leeper connection between EMF and childhood leukemia.

David L Strayer

Professor, Psychology Department, University of Utah, USA and principal author of the Transport Research study

Dimitris Panagopoulos

Research Scientist, Department of Biology University of Athens, Athens, Greece; and the Radiation and Environmental Biophysics Research Centre, Athens. Author of 'Electromagnetic Interaction between Environmental Fields and Living Systems Determines Health and Well-Being.'

Dominique Belpomme

Professor of clinical oncology, University Paris-Descartes; president Association for Research and Treatment against Cancer (ARTAC); chairman of International Society of Doctors for Environment, France (ISDE)

Franz Adlkofer

Executive director, VERUM-Foundation for Behaviour and Environment, Munich, Germany; chairman, Pandora Foundation (promotion of free and independent science and research); lead scientist of the EU-funded REFLEX research programme (1999–2004)

George Carlo
Epidemiologist and public health scientist with over thirty years of experience and an extensive list of medical, scientific, and public policy publications; has served on many federal and state government commissions and advisory panels; chief scientist and lead epidemiologist, Wireless Technology Research (1993–1999); chairman, Science and Public Policy Institute, Washington DC (non-profit)

Gerald Hyland
Former associate fellow, Department of Physics, University of Warwick, UK; executive member, International Institute of Biophysics, Neuss-Holzheim, Germany; member of International Commission for Electromagnetic Safety (ICEMS)

Gerd Oberfeld
Head of Environmental Health and Medicine Public Health Department, Salzburg; special interest is environmental medicine; advisor to and speaker for Environmental Medicine for the Austrian Medical Association, Vienna, Austria; organizer of the 2000 International Conference for Cell Tower Siting - Linking Science and Public Health

Joel M Moskowitz
Director, Center for Family and Community Health, University of California, Berkeley, USA. Research interests are health promotion and disease prevention, health effects of mobile phones.

Kjell Hansson Mild
Biologist; currently conducting research on bioeffects of electromagnetic fields as associate professor in medical physics, Department of Radiation Physics, University of Umea, Sweden; previously adjunct professor at Orebro University; board member of the European Bioelectromagnetics Association; co-authored the BioInitiative Report section on brain tumors and acoustic neuromas.

Leif Salford
Professor and chairman, Department of Neurosurgery at Lund University, Sweden; former president of the Swedish Neurosurgical Association

Lennart Hardell
Professor of oncology and cancer epidemiology at University Hospital, Orebro, Sweden; recent research - the use of cellular and cordless telephones and the risk for brain tumours; co-authored the BioInitiative Report section on brain tumors and acoustic neuromas; among the first to associate dioxins with increased cancer risk; member of International Commission for Electromagnetic Safety (ICEMS)

Levi Schächter
Professor, Department of Electrical Engineering, Israel Institute of Technology, Haifa, Israel. One of his main areas of research is the interaction of electromagnetic fields with the human body.

Lukas H Margaritis

Research scientist specializing in radiation biology-effects of non-ionizing radiation; professor emeritus, cell biology, radiobiology and electron microscopy, University of Athens, Greece

Martin Blank

Associate professor, Department of Physiology and Cellular Biophysics, Columbia University, New York, USA (retired after over forty years of research and teaching); author, the BioInitiative Report's Section 7 on stress response; editor of the 2009 issue of *Pathophysiology* on EMF. His specialty has been research into the effects of EMF on cell biochemistry and cell membrane function.

Michael Kundi

Professor and head, Institute of Environmental Health, University of Vienna, Austria; member of several standards committees, including Committee on Electromagnetic fields; author of the BioInitiative Report section on the evidence for childhood cancers (Leukaemia); co-authored the Report section on brain tumors and acoustic neuromas

Neil Cherry (1946–2003)

Biophysicist; associate professor, Environmental Health, Lincoln University, New Zealand. Professional scientific background in biology, physics, biophysics, and environmental epidemiology.

Olle Johansson

Research scientist specializing in the field of EMF radiation and its biological and health effects, particularly in relation to electrical hypersensitivity; associate professor and head of the Experimental Dermatology Unit, Department of Neuroscience, Karolinska Institute, Stockholm, Sweden; author of the BioInitiative Report section on the immune system

Om Gandhi

Professor of electrical and computer engineering, University of Utah, USA; has chaired committees on RF standards and the health effects of RF; author of *Biological Effects and Medical Applications of Electromagnetic Energy*

Örjan Hallberg

Research scientist specializing in the field of EMF radiation and its biological and health effects; formerly working for decades as quality and environmental manager within Ericsson, then as researcher with the Department of Neuroscience, Karolinska Institute, Stockholm, Sweden; currently with Hallberg Independent Research

Ross Adey (1922–2004)

Former professor of neurology, Loma Linda University School of Medicine, USA; served on White House Advisory Committees; addressed Congress; chair of the National Council on Radiation Committee on ELF's

Siegal Sadetzki
Epidemiologist and physician; Israeli Health Ministry senior advisor on cell phone effects; senior lecturer, Sackler Faculty of Medicine, Department of Epidemiology and Preventative Medicine, Tel Aviv University, Israel

Vini G Khurana
Associate professor of neurosurgery, Australian National University Medical School, ACT; staff specialist neurosurgeon, The Canberra Hospital, ACT, Australia; visiting attending neurosurgeon, Royal Melbourne Hospital, VIC, Australia; author, *Brain Surgery* and *The Brain Aneurysm*

Yuri Grigoriev
Research scientist; chairman of Russian National Committee on Non-Ionizing Radiation Protection, Moscow, Russian Federation; member of the International Advising Committee on WHO EMF Project; board member of *Journal of Radiation Biology and Ecology*

2   *The Electrical Engineers*

> ➢   *Those with extensive qualifications and experience in the field of electrical engineering, who have specialised in RF Radiation and cell phones, and their biological effects and impact on human health*

Alasdair Philips
Founder of Powerwatch UK; has a background in both electrical and electronic engineering; member of the SAGE, the UK Department of Health's committee into radiation's effect on health; member of the UK Health Protection Agency's EMF Discussion Group; co-author, *Cellphones and Brain Tumors: 15 Reasons for Concern.*

L Lloyd Morgan
Director, Central Brain Tumor Registry of the United States; senior research fellow, Environmental Health Trust; scientific advisor, EM Radiation Research Trust; volunteer with the National Brain Tumor Foundation; primary author, *Cellphones and Brain Tumors: 15 Reasons for Concern*

Vicki Warren
Former executive director and program director of the Institute of Building Biology and Ecology (IBE) USA; electrical engineer with vast experience working within the power industry; BBEC-trained through the IBE, and CERSA-certified through the Safe Wireless Initiative. As director of Wings of Eagle Healthy Living, she helps others protect their health from exposure to electromagnetic radiation.

3   The Public Advocates

➢   *Scientists who have compiled opinion or advocacy summaries of science addressing RF radiation/cell phones, and published their findings and opinions at conferences or in the open media*

➢   *Scientists who have been quoted on their opinion of mobile telecommunications*

➢   *Non-scientists who have compiled their own advocacy summaries of the research into RF radiation/cell phones in order to educate and inform the general public*

Annie Sasco
Epidemiologist and physician, president of HealthCam; manages the team of epidemiologists for Cancer Prevention within the Institute of Pubic Health, Epidemiology and Development, Bordeaux, France. Her career has been focussed on the study of cancer in a globalized environment.

B Blake Levitt
Award-winning journalist, writing about the fields of medicine and science with a special interest in non-ionizing radiation; author, *Electromagnetic Fields: A Consumer's Guide to the Issue and How to Protect Ourselves*; editor, *Cell Towers: Wireless Convenience? or Environmental Hazard?*

Camilla Rees
Health care advocate; CEO, Wide Angle Health, USA. Launched 'Campaign for Radiation Free Schools' and 'EMF Help Blog'; co-author, *Public Health SOS: The Shadow Side of the Wireless Revolution*; co-author, *Cellphones and Brain Tumors: 15 Reasons for Concern.*

Cindy Sage
Environmental consultant and public policy researcher since 1982; owner of Sage & Associates, environmental consulting firm in California, USA; founder of the BioInitiative Working Group; co-chair of the Collaborative for Health and the Environment EMF Working Group; co-editor of the BioInitiative Report (2007 and 2012) and author of several of their sections

Devra Lee Davis
Epidemiologist; director, Center on Environmental Oncology, University of Pittsburgh Cancer Institute, USA; professor, Department of Epidemiology, Graduate School of Health, University of Pittsburgh

Don Maisch
Researcher, founder of EMF Facts Consultancy; author of many papers on the subject of EMR, cell phones and RF

Gene Barnett
Director of the Brain Tumor and Neuro-Oncology Center, Cleveland Clinic, USA; vice chairman, Department of Neurological Surgery. He has a special interest in neuro-oncology; is on a number of editorial boards; and is a reviewer for neurosurgery journals.

Ian Gibson
Biologist and cancer specialist for forty years; honorary Fellow of the British Association of Science; former chair of Science and Technology Select Committee, the Parliamentary, Scientific Committee, and the Parliamentary Office of Science and Technology; dean of the School of Biological Sciences, University of East Anglia. He was three times elected as MP for Norwich North in the UK.

Larry Rosen
Research psychologist and computer educator; past chair and professor of psychology at California State University.

Lawrence Challis
Emeritus professor of Physics, University of Nottingham, UK; vice-chairman of the Stewart Committee (British government investigation in to mobile phones in 2000); awarded the OBE in 1996 for services to scientific research.

Olga Naidenko
Senior scientist, Environmental Working Group, US; researcher into molecular and structural immunology; author, *Limit Your Exposure to Cell Phone Radiation.*

Paul J Rosch
Clinical professor of medicine and psychiatry, New York Medical College, New York, USA; Chairman of the board, the American Institute of Stress; honorary vice-president of the International Stress Management Association, and chairman of its US branch. Recipient of many honours and awards, he has written extensively over the past forty-five years on the role of stress in health and illness, including serving as editor and on the editorial board of several publications.

Sarah Starkey
UK neuroscientist with a particular interest in wireless systems in schools.

4   *The others with experience relevant to this field*

➤   *Professionals with experience in related and relevant fields who offer their opinions in order to educate and inform the general public*

Carl Hilliard
Consumer advocate and litigating attorney who specialized in telecommunications law and acquisitions; former associate professor of law, California Western School of Law, University of California; pursued consumer protection efforts against wireless carriers for a $1 billion settlement for consumers; president of Wireless Consumers Alliance; former mayor of Del Mar, California.

Chris Woollams
CEO and founder of CANCERactive, UK; presents worldwide on cancer and cancer prevention; editor, *Integrated Cancer and Oncology News* (*icon* magazine).

Elizabeth Barris
Founder and director, The People's Initiative Foundation; co-author, *Cellphones and Brain Tumors: 15 Reasons for Concern*. She submitted *The Children's Wireless Protection Act*, calling for warning labels and for the need to replace Wi-Fi in schools with hard-wiring.

Erik Huber
Environmental spokesman for the Doctor's Chamber for Vienna.

Michael Lerner
President and founder of non-profit Commonweal, Washington DC, USA.

Nicholas Negroponte
Architect and computer scientist; founder and former director of Massachusetts Institute of Technology, Media Laboratory; founder and chairman of non-profit One Laptop per Child.

Thomas Rau
Founder and chief medical director, Paracelus Klinik, Switzerland.

It should be made clear that - with only a few exceptions - the experts listed above did not in any way collaborate on this book. They have been included because they have, at some point in time, made on-the-record comments that are particularly relevant to the subject matter, and help to illustrate and clarify the information being passed on here.

There are also those quoted in this book who have not been included in its companion, 'Hold The Phone'. Inclusion relates not only to professional standing, but also to the relevance of the quotes to the material. The fact that someone is missing from this list is not intended to infer that they are not a credible authority within their field.

There are also some listed here who do not stand out as being 'big names'. Because they are busy 'doing the work' they often fly under the radar, and you may never be aware of the important contributions they have made. They are the real deal: the unsung heroes in all of this.

Please note that there are only very brief details given here for each person. This in no way reflects the total career of, or contributions made by, each of these individuals. Each précis is merely intended to give the reader a brief insight into the depth of their experience, and highlight why their quotes are important and relevant to the subject of this book.

These quotes are included as it was felt that they were in line with the intent of this book, namely, to provide education about this highly newsworthy subject. The aim is also to encourage readers to extend their own knowledge and research, through investigating further the named sources and resources.

These quotes have been freely available for all to see in newspapers, magazines, TV, radio, books, DVDs, open letters, reports, studies, articles, submissions and testimonials, statements and proceedings, blogs, newsletters, and other sources that are easily accessible on the Internet. They are fully referenced in the back of the book.

A WORD ON "EXPERTS"

I am always cautious when I hear the word *"expert"*. It is a term that has lost some of its credibility due to overuse by the media, and because it's often self-proclaimed. My main caution, however, is due to the effect the word seems to have on us.

Like gurus, experts can be disempowering; and by that I mean that we can be tempted to hand our power over to them. "They know more, so they can make the decisions". Also, simply by believing that they know more, we can belittle ourselves. In our own minds this can translate to "If they are more, surely that means we must be less?"

In adopting someone else's viewpoint, in trusting them, we sometimes override our own instincts and intuition. We trust them more than we trust ourselves. In cutting ourselves off from our intuition, the vital guiding light in our lives, we leave ourselves open to floundering rudderless in a sea of never-ending information.

When it comes to *your* life, *you* are the expert. While it is important and informative to listen to the voice of others, you need to follow that up by being finely tuned into to your own inner voice: your intuition.

The quotes in this book are all from genuine experts in their field: credible, experienced, and professional. Their information is here to help you. However, as when you read any advice or information, read it not only with your eyes and mind but also with your 'gut'. Even though what you're reading may seem hard to believe at first, at times confronting or even a little overwhelming, check in with yourself to see how you really feel about it.

- ➢ Does what is presented here make sense to you?
- ➢ Does it resonate somewhere deep inside?
- ➢ Does it feel as if it might just be right?
- ➢ Do you feel urged to take action, no matter how quiet and gentle that little inner voice?

If so, then please listen to *yourself,* and take the warnings on board.

Part 1

Phones and Wireless

How you can protect your health

Phones and Wireless 101
The Basics

"Men occasionally stumble over the truth,
but most of them pick themselves up and hurry off
as if nothing ever happened."

Winston Churchill

SOME FACTS ABOUT CELL PHONES, CORDLESS PHONES, AND WIRELESS

We have never witnessed anything quite as phenomenal as the uptake of wireless technology. Its growth has been truly exponential.

In only six years, the number of cell phone accounts in the market increased from two billion in 2006 to a staggering six billion in 2012. Some predict that to reach 7 billion in 2013.

From Asia to America, and everywhere in between, it's safe to say that only a tiny percentage of individuals are free from exposure to communications technology networks. In fact, some countries are now opting to phase out landline phones completely and will offer only mobile phone connectivity.

This is a situation that, whether we've chosen to opt in or not, now affects us all.

Here are the priorities about mobiles phones and wireless:

➢ Mobile phones, cordless phones, and 'wireless' devices *all* work using microwave radiation (which lies within the broader range of radiofrequency radiation, or RFR).

➢ They all also *emit* microwave radiation.

➢ In 2011 the WHO officially declared this radiation "a possible human carcinogen".

➢ There are many, many, *many* research studies that show that microwave radiation and RFR can alter biology, and have the potential to significantly affect health.

➤   Some of this research evidence links exposure to microwave radiation/RFR with:

- alterations to both brain function and heart function
- changes in behaviour
- impairment of immune system function
- changes in biological and genetic structure, and damage to DNA
- inhibition of the body's ability to *repair* damaged DNA
- interference with the quality and quantity of sperm, reducing fertility
- alterations to the brain, including pathological leakage of the blood brain barrier
- disruption of fetal brain development
- reduced quality of sleep, impaired melatonin production
- a wide range of health disorders, from headaches to brain cancer

➤   Children are especially vulnerable to, and affected by, exposure to microwave radiation. (It is linked to learning difficulties, hyperactivity, behavioural issues, ADD, autism, and childhood leukaemia.)

➤   The radiation from phones and wireless appliances affects more than just the people using them. They, and the antennae and routers that power them, emit high levels of radiation: *passive* radiation that envelops everyone around them.

➤   Passive smoking can be avoided by closing a door, but passive radiation from phones and wireless can't. It passes right through doors, windows, walls, and ceilings.

➤   Because microwave radiation is invisible, and most can't feel it, people are generally unaware that they're exposed to it.

- Based on current research, many governments and health experts around the world have issued official warnings to the public, advising them to reduce their exposure to mobile phones, cordless phones, and Wi-Fi.

- The media reports saying the "jury is still out" on the safety of cell phones can give a false sense of security. There are *thousands* of studies that have found evidence of the potential to affect both biology and health. Then there are studies that have failed to find an effect.

- Despite what you may hear or read, remember: Research that fails to *find* an effect is **not** the same thing as research that proves there is *no* effect! Absence of proof is not proof of absence. Because of this, no one can tell you that it's safe to use a mobile phone.

The Good News: There *are* ways you can help to protect your health by reducing your exposure to microwave radiation.

This book will show you *how* to do just that.

All great truths begin as blasphemies."

George Bernard Shaw

> *"The world's largest biological experiment ever, takes place since few years . . .*
>
> *and now one third of the world's population is included in the experiment as test persons, voluntarily exposing their brains to electromagnetic fields produced by their mobile phones.*
>
> *The other two thirds constitute a control group, however not ideal, as many of the non-users are exposed to 'passive mobile phoning' and other types of radio frequency radiation."*
>
> **Leif Salford** (2006) **(3)**
>
> *(Said in 2006: There are now over 6 billion mobile phone subscribers)*

"There are only two mistakes one can make along the road to truth: not going all the way, and not starting."

Buddha

RECENT DISCOVERIES

WHO declares Radiofrequency Radiation as a Class 2B "Possible Human Carcinogen"

Lyon, France, May 31, 2011 – The WHO/International Agency for Research on Cancer (IARC) has classified radiofrequency electromagnetic fields as possibly carcinogenic to humans (Group 2B), based on an increased risk for glioma, a malignant type of brain cancer associated with wireless phone use.

From May 24-31 2011, a Working Group of 31 scientists from 14 countries has been meeting at IARC in Lyon, France, to assess the potential carcinogenic hazards from exposure to radiofrequency electromagnetic fields.

Conclusions: Dr Jonathan Samet (University of Southern California, USA), overall Chairman of the Working Group, indicated that "the evidence, while still accumulating, is strong enough to support a conclusion and the 2B classification. The conclusion means that there could be some risk, and therefore we need to keep a close watch for a link between cell phones and cancer risk."

"Given the potential consequences for public health of this classification and findings," said IARC Director Christopher Wild, "it is important that additional research be conducted into the long–term, heavy use of mobile phones. Pending the availability of such information, it is important to take pragmatic measures to reduce exposure such as hands–free devices or texting."

WHO/IARC, May 2011 (4)

Comments on the IARC Class 2B Rating: "Possible Human Carcinogen"

"In the end of May 2011 . . . IARC of the WHO in Lyon classified RF electromagnetic fields, to which wireless radiation belongs, as "possibly carcinogenic".

Results from basic research with proven changes in structure and functions of genes after the exposure of isolated human and animal cells, but also from exposed animals itself, that would have lent weight to the epidemiological observations were, however, not all considered.

Had these results been taken into account according to their significance, the classification would not have been "possibly carcinogenic" but rather "probably carcinogenic"."

Franz Adlkofer *(2011)* *(5)*

"The existing science is very clear there is risk of cancer from cell phone use.

*The warning might have been 2A (**probable** human carcinogen) if there were a larger number of animal studies showing this, or if there were a larger number of up-to-date human studies.*

It's important to recognize the Interphone study on which the classification to a large extent relied was completed in 2004, and current studies reflecting usage patterns today would be far more damning, possibly earning a Class 1 "Human Carcinogen".

Alasdair Philips *(2011)* *(6)*

> "The US government now has a scientific basis to issue precautionary health warnings, revise existing cell phone regulations and fund research on radio frequency electromagnetic field radiation.
>
> A $1 per year fee on each cell phone would generate $300 million annually for research and education."
>
> **Joel Moskowitz** (7)

"We know the truth, not only by the reason, but also by the heart."

Blaise Pascal

Cell and Mobile Phones

Quick Tips

What are the issues, and what to do?

"Every convenience brings its own inconveniences along with it."

Proverb

CELL PHONES AT A GLANCE: THE ISSUES

Cell phones and mobile phones emit microwave radiation.

Mobile phone use is linked to brain tumours, and a variety of chronic health conditions.

Mobile phone use can also affect your:

➢ sleep,

➢ memory,

➢ brain function,

➢ moods and behaviour,

➢ immune system,

➢ fertility, and

➢ ability to feel well, healthy, and full of vitality.

Children are especially vulnerable to radiation during mobile phone calls. Radiation from a phone can penetrate through almost the entire brain of a young child.

Pregnant women using mobile phones risk affecting their unborn child. Research has shown behavioural and learning difficulties later in life for these children.

"People who sell mobile phones are making a positive assertion of safety: there is no risk.

That just cannot be done."

Cindy Sage (2000) **(88)**

Please Note:

The terms 'radiofrequency radiation', 'microwave radiation' and 'information carrying radio waves' will all be used throughout the book - often interchangeably.

All technical terms within this book have been deliberately generalised to keep the information as simple and accessible as possible, and to prevent it from getting bogged down by technicality and detail.

For those who do wish to have more precise information on each term and frequency range, please search the plethora of information on the Internet for "radiofrequency radiation" and the other terms used.

Please also remember that the research quoted and highlighted here is providing us with a link to potential effects. It is not a foregone conclusion that these effects will happen.

We are all individuals, and because we're not all the same our responses vary quite markedly. It appears that we differ in:

➢ *whether we're affected*

➢ *what affects us*

➢ *how much we're affected, and*

➢ *the ways in which we're affected*

Cell Phone Safety Tips

What to do then?

How to protect your health?

*The following are the priorities you need to know
about mobile phones
and what you can do to minimise
your exposure to their radiation.*

*"The saddest aspect of life right now
is that science gathers knowledge
faster than society gathers wisdom."*

Isaac Asimov

CELL PHONES - SAFETY TIP # 1

1. The absolute priority
Keep the phone away from your head

In order for mobile phones to work, mobile telecommunications technology 'sprays' microwave radiation into the air so that you can pick up a signal wherever you go. As soon as your mobile phone is in use, it too starts 'spraying' radiation. If you're in contact with it, the radiation goes into you.

The sphere of the most intense radiation around a phone is called a 'near-field plume'. During an 'average' phone call, this is estimated to be roughly eight to twelve inches (20–30 cm) in diameter. When the phone is next to your ear, that plume of intense radiation penetrates right through your skull, and goes directly 4 in/10 cm deep into your brain's soft tissue.

> This microwave radiation can change the cellular structure of our brains.

> It can also change the electrical activity of our brains: the way in which they work and communicate with the rest of our body.

> Holding a mobile phone next to your head for long periods of time is linked through significant research with the occurrence and growth of brain tumours.

"Mobile companies hide the figures on how much radiation they give off in the back of manuals . . . But modern phones give out 217 electromagnetic pulses every second into your head."

Alasdair Philips (2009) **(9)**

> "Recent epidemiologic studies of adults from those few nations where cell phone use has been extensive for a decade or longer indicate significantly increased risk of a variety of brain tumors."
>
> **Guiliani L, Soffritti M** (2010) **(10)**
>
> Research study: Guiliani L, Soffritti M. Non-Thermal effects and mechanisms of interaction between electromagnetic fields and living matter

CELL PHONES - SAFETY TIPS # 2

2.   Use an earpiece, headset, or handset

The whole idea of using these is to try to get the radiation that's coming out of the phone as far away from your brain as possible.

Using an earpiece (wired or airtube ones are preferable) *while holding the phone away from you* also prevents the radiation from being absorbed into your body.

> "The headset is the best interim remedy, because it gives you the opportunity - it empowers you - to take the radiation away from your body, and still use the phone."
>
> **George Carlo** (2005) **(11)**

Plug-in handsets are a great idea. Looking like the handle of a retro phone, they plug into most cell phones. They enable you to keep the radiation well away from your head - and if the phone is kept at a distance, away from your body too.

Leaving one of these on your desk, or wherever else you make most of your calls, will mean it's immediately to hand whenever you need to use the phone.

Once you've made a habit of keeping it plugged in, you won't even need to think about it. Just this one small change in behaviour will prevent a tremendous amount of radiation entering into the soft tissue of your brain.

Whatever new devices come onto the market – however enticing the appeal of their marketing - **avoid putting *anything* that uses wireless technology anywhere near your head.**

CELL PHONES - SAFETY TIPS # 3

3.   *Use Bluetooth earpieces and headsets with caution*

During a call a Bluetooth headset emits less radiation than a phone, so using one is preferable to putting the phone right next to your ear. However, it still exposes the cells of your head and brain to radiation.

When a Bluetooth headset is switched on, it is continually in communication with your phone (and other Bluetooth devices): they stay in touch with each other by constantly 'pinging' or signalling back and forth. When this happens, it's not only the phone but also the headset that is emitting microwave radiation.

If you 'wear' the earpiece all day, then your entire bioelectrical system faces the challenge of constant interference from the radiation. As the earpiece is on your head, there is the risk that this can affect your brain.

Because of this, if for some reason you *have* to use one, they are best used only while you're actually making the call, and only for short periods. Take it off as soon as you've finished. (Airtube or wired earpieces are a safer option.)

CELL PHONES - SAFETY TIP # 4

4. *Use the loudspeaker*

Using the phone's loudspeaker, or speakerphone function, is another excellent option. It's cheaper than an earpiece and doesn't take as much fiddling around when a call comes in.

Using the loudspeaker, *whilst holding the phone away from you* (or putting it on a desk), presents the smallest chance possible of any radiation crossing into your head or body.

However, If you are going to use the loudspeaker, please think of those around you: find a quiet spot where you're not going to disturb anyone.

CELL PHONES - SAFETY TIP # 5

5.   Use an online phone service to make calls

Using your computer - as long as it's a cable-connected computer - to make calls via an online phone service such as Skype can dramatically cut down your exposure to radiation.

"And if I hold it to my head like this, there is no way that I can avoid getting a sizeable amount of that energy in my head and my hand.

This is the first generation that has put relatively high-powered transmitters against the head day after day after day.

The picture that's emerging is that, over the lifetime of the individual, you may see changes that could be considered health effects or potential health risks."

Ross Adey (2000) **(14)**

CELL PHONES - SAFETY TIP # 6

6.   Keep changing sides

If you have to place the phone next to your ear, then make absolutely sure that it's not kept next to the same ear all the time.

Research, especially the long-term studies, point to a clear link between the amount of time a phone has been used and brain cancer. The longer a phone has been held against the ear, the greater the risk. It also shows that the more the phone is used *on one side of the head*, the greater the risk of cancer occurring within *that side* of the brain.

There is good news. Alternating the side of the head to which you hold the phone has been shown to *significantly* reduce this risk.

> *"The uncertainty about the relationship between the use of mobile phones (MPs) and the increase of head tumour risk can be solved by a critical analysis of the methodological elements of both the positive and the negative studies.*
>
> *Results by Hardell indicate a cause/effect relationship: exposures for or latencies from ≥ 10 years to MPs increase by up to 100% the risk of tumour on the same side of the head preferred for phone use (ipsilateral tumours) - which is the only one significantly irradiated. . ."*
>
> *"However, also in the Interphone studies a clear and statistically significant increase of ipsilateral head tumours (gliomas, neuromas and parotid gland tumours) is quite common in people having used MPs since or for ≥ 10 years."*
>
> **Levis AG et al** (2011) (15)
>
> Research Study: Levis AG et al. *Mobile phones and head tumours: it is time to read and highlight data in a proper way.*

CELL PHONES - SAFETY TIP # 7

7.   Keep it brief

For the radiation from a mobile phone to have an effect on your biology, there needs to be a *sustained* exposure to the signal.

Unfortunately, 'sustained' is not as long as you may think. According to Dr George Carlo, that is anything over *twenty seconds*. What that means is that any call lasting more than twenty seconds may cause biological disruption to your body.

A recent Japanese study found significant risk for those who used mobile phones for more than twenty minutes a day for at least five years: three times more acoustic neuromas than could be expected. *(See below)*.

Tumour location was linked to the side of phone use.

> "*A significantly increased risk was identified for mobile phone use for >20 min/day on average.*"
>
> **Sato Y et al** *(2010)* *(16)*
> *Research Study: Sato Y et al. A case-case study of mobile phone use and acoustic neuroma risk in Japan*

Because of this, keep all your calls as brief as you can. If someone calls you, say that you'll call back on a landline (a *corded* one.)

> "*Remember, you have perhaps 2,000 minutes (cumulative lifetime) before you are in the heavy user category and at statistically significantly increased risk for glioma.*"
>
> **Cindy Sage** *(2009)* *(17)*

CELL PHONES - SAFETY TIP # 8

8. Practice 'safe text'
Text instead of calling

Texting helps you to keep the phone, and its radiation, away from your head.

A text (because it's sent using only a short burst of power) also involves far less radiation than a call.

Make sure you hold the phone away from you when you're texting.

> (Re: children using mobile phones)
>
> *"The Stewart report recommended that they should not use them to any extent.*
>
> *I think the advice to secondary school children is to use them sparingly, to text rather than phone, given the uncertainty."*
>
> **Lawrence Challis** *(2009)* *(18)*

7.8 trillion SMS messages were sent in 2011.

This is expected to reach 9.6 trillion in 2015.

CELL PHONES - SAFETY TIP # 9

9.   *When your phone is connecting to another phone - Keep it well away from you*

When your phone is trying to make a connection with another phone, it uses far more power than it does once the connection is established. This need for more power results in your phone emitting far more radiation.

If you are holding the phone next to your ear whilst the connection is being made, then these higher levels of radiation are going straight into your brain.

While making a connection, the phone emits not only far higher levels of radiation, but the cloud of radiation that surrounds the phone extends over a much larger area, which also goes on to affect those around you.

10. When there's a weak signal (low signal bars) - Keep it away from you

A 'low' signal indicates that there is limited reception in the area you're in, and your phone will have to work much harder to make contact with the base station.

This also means that it will require more power, which will increase the amount of radiation that's emitted from it.

> "The higher the tower strength - the more signal bars you have - the less energy your cell phone must generate to maintain communication."
>
> **Vicki Warren** (2010) **(19)**

This is particularly relevant in sparsely populated areas, such as country regions, where signal strength is frequently weak.

> "Mobile phones can use up to 1,000 times more power when they are far away from a base station.
>
> Those using cell phones in rural areas at a distance from the transmitter absorb far more energy from the handset."
>
> **Kjell Hansson Mild** (2009) **(20)**

CELL PHONES - SAFETY TIP # 11

11.   When you're inside a metal structure
Avoid using your phone

When mobile phones are used inside a metal structure, such as planes, trains, and cars, they usually have to work harder to make a connection.

As we've seen, this extra 'work' means that you're exposed to more radiation than usual if you're using the phone inside one of these.

ALSO, microwave radiation is reflected by metal. This means that the metal walls of the car, plane, or train make it harder for the radiation to escape. Instead, it can keep bouncing around inside (which is the principle behind the microwave oven).

Whether you're the one using the phone, or you're just sitting close to someone else who is, you're being caught up in a cloud of microwave radiation that's making your transport act like your oven.

This information is really important for anyone whose work means that they constantly have to use their phones while they're on the road.

> *"It varies from model to model, but in general when a cell phone is being used in a full-strength signal area, the signal from the cell phone can have a potential impact on anyone within approximately 6 feet (2 meters) of the cell phone.*
>
> *As the signal strength decreases, and therefore the cell phone strength increases, this distance increases proportionally.*
>
> *The actual distance of effect depends entirely on the direction and magnitude of the signal and whether the signal transmission is occurring within an enclosed area where there is significant reflection, such as an airplane, car or train."*
>
> **Vicki Warren** *(2010)* *(22)*

CELL PHONES - SAFETY TIP # 12

12. *When you're travelling at speed - Avoid using your phone*

When you're moving at high speed in a car or train, your phone has to struggle hard to locate the nearest antenna and then connect to it.

This creates electrical 'surging' as the phone regularly 'pulses' while it tries to make contact with the nearest antenna.

Because you're constantly changing position, it has to do this repeatedly, and often. All this hard work increases the power levels of the phone, often to its maximum, increasing the radiation levels.

This increases in high-use areas (like cities) as your connection is moved from antenna to antenna according to the available capacity.

This is especially true when you're in a car, moving quickly from one area to another.

The other reason not to use mobile phones in cars is that it dramatically increases the chances of having an accident.

Much of the research has made the observation that crashes are due to distraction, and drivers' lack of concentration when using phones.

Given what we know about microwave radiation exposure and its effect on the brain's ability to function properly, perhaps we should also be looking at whether it is the radiation emitted by the phones that is affecting the brain's inability to concentrate.

Is it possible that the accidents are a consequence, not just of inattention, but also of the mobile phone's interference with brain function?

> *"If you put a 20-year-old driver behind the wheel with a cell phone, his reaction times are the same as a 70-year-old driver.*
>
> *It's like instantly ageing a large number of drivers."*
>
> **David Strayer** *(2005)* *(23)*

Cell Phones - Safety Tip # 13

13. *Have a car kit fitted*

If you do need to make calls in your car, have a special external car aerial fitted, along with a hands-free kit. This will prevent you from needing to hold the phone, and also minimises the amount of radiation inside your car.

Be aware that Bluetooth uses wireless, which still relies on filling the air inside your car with radiation.

If you have a Bluetooth feature in your car, you can reduce your exposure by turning it off when you're not actually on the phone.

> *"Due to the available health effects research results of low level long-term nonionizing radiation exposure, and since more than four billion people now are using mobile phones, the Precautionary Principle should be adopted promptly for these issues. . . .*
>
> *People should be advised to reduce RF/MW exposure, for example using head phones and hands-free kits until new technologies or new health effect research results are available."*
>
> **Alvaro Augusto A de Salles** *(24)*

CELL PHONES - SAFETY TIP # 14

14. *Avoid using your phone*
- when it is damaged

Mobile phones that have been damaged can have problems picking up a signal, or connecting to other phones.

This leads to more power being used, again meaning that more radiation is emitted.

> *"Damaged cell phones and PDA's (dropped, banged around) often have much higher emissions. Make sure if one is issued to you, it is in good condition.*
>
> **Cindy Sage** *(2009) (25)*

CELL PHONES - SAFETY TIP # 15

15. Avoid 'wearing' your phone

If you have a phone that's capable of downloading data, such as emails, web pages, music or videos, be aware that this can create dramatic surges of very powerful radiation.

If you're 'wearing' your phone by carrying it around on your body, then very high levels of radiation are going into your body each time these surges or downloads happen. Frequent downloads mean that you can face the risk of being constantly irradiated, potentially leading to chronic exposure levels.

Even when your phone isn't in use, it has to intermittently signal back and forth to the antenna to let it know that it's there, ready and waiting for the next call.

This signalling appears as 'noise', which can disrupt the body's bioelectric system, especially communication between the brain and body, pulsing of the heart, and functioning of cells.

Studies have found biological effects even when the phone is in 'stand-by' mode.

> "The electromagnetic radiation causes cells to change in a way that makes them cancer forming."
>
> "It can increase the risk of cancer two to five times."
>
> **Neil Cherry (26)**

Mobile phone companies are well aware of this and cover themselves by giving a warning, usually somewhere towards the back of the phone instruction books.

Be aware that phones are often carried next to important organs, such as the:

➢ liver (on the belt),

➢ kidneys (back of the belt)

➢ reproductive organs, (jean pockets) and

➢ heart (shirt pocket).

> *"When you have the phone in your pocket, or if you have it on your belt, you're exposing other important areas.*
>
> *Now you know, 80% of our red blood cells are formed in the flat bones of the hip. So that, when you have your phone on your belt, you're exposing the bone that makes your blood. That's not good."*
>
> **George Carlo** *(2005)* *(27)*

There has been a disturbing increase in the incidence of young women carrying their mobile phones around tucked inside their bra.

Apart from the danger of disruption to the electrical system of the heart, there is also the potential for harm to those other delicate areas that the phone is close to: the lungs, the lymph system, and particularly the soft tissue of the breast itself.

> *"Cells in the body react to EMFs as potentially harmful, just like to other environmental toxins, including heavy metals and toxic chemicals. The DNA in living cells recognizes electromagnetic fields at very low levels of exposure; and produces a biochemical stress response."*
>
> **Martin Blank** *(2007)* *(28)*

There are a few 'wearable' communication accessories being marketed at the moment. And there will be more in the future. For the sake of your health please think really, really carefully about their implications.

16. Boys, keep your phone out of your pockets

Infertility in men has been linked to their use of mobile phones, particularly if they carry them on their body. It's very common for phones to be carried in the front pockets of jeans.

The phone is then resting next to their groin, allowing the radiation to permeate into their testicles.

> ". . . .Australia's John Aitken is saying the issue "deserves our immediate attention". In a new study, Aitken has reported that cell phone radiation damages human sperm - as well as DNA.
>
> Cell phone use and radiation has now been shown to harm sperm in five different countries, including by two different groups in the United States, one of which is at the Cleveland Clinic.
>
> Aitken's message is simple: "Men who want to have children should not keep active mobile phones in their trouser pocket"."
>
> **Microwave News** (2009) **(29)**

There are many studies showing how exposure to electromagnetic and microwave radiation reduces sperm count and sperm quality, which poses risks to both the chances of getting pregnant, and the health of the future child.

Studies also link RFR to testicular cancer. There has apparently been an 'epidemic increase in the US' in the cases of very young men developing testicular cancer.

> *"Mobile companies hide the figures on how much radiation they give off in the back of manuals . . . Males should not keep them in a pocket because they drastically affect fertility."*
>
> *Alasdair Philips* (2009) *(30)*

There is even a study showing that this radiation is magnified by metal objects such as coins, rings, and zips.

There is no doubt that it's best for men, and even young boys, to avoid putting the phones into their pockets.

CELL PHONES - SAFETY TIP # 17

17. Girls, keep your phones away from your pelvis

Not much research regarding female fertility has been released so far. However, the latest studies do indicate an effect on the ovaries.

An important factor to remember is that unlike sperm production, which is a continual process, women's eggs are formed whilst they are in utero and then carried inside them from birth.

Women constantly carrying phones close to their ovaries are likely to be running the risk of exposing their eggs to chronic levels of radiation.

Early indications from research on animals show that there is the potential for an inhibiting effect on females' ability to reproduce. Unfortunately, it's also possible that these reproductive deficiencies can be passed on to their daughters.

Exposure to cell phone/radiofrequency radiation has also been linked to increased incidence of miscarriage.

It's fair to say that the picture painted by research already indicates that close exposure is best avoided for women. As a precaution, they are particularly advised not to carry phones anywhere near their reproductive organs.

Effects on Fertility

"There have been several studies showing that mobile phone use reduces male fertility. One of the more recent (1) showed that using a mobile phone for more than four hours a day caused a reduction in sperm numbers, motility and viability, each of around 25 percent.

Effects on female fertility have not yet been studied but, since all the eggs that a woman will ever have were already in her ovaries before she was born, the cumulative effect could be considerable."

Andrew Goldsworthy (2009) (31)

CELL PHONES - SAFETY TIP # 18

18. If you have to keep your phone on your body - Make sure it's 'back to front'

It's important to remember that with some phones, more radiation comes *out of the back* of the phone than the front.

So, if for some reason you do have to carry a phone on you, make sure that you place the back of the phone *facing away* from your body.

CELL PHONES - SAFETY TIP # 19

19. *Minimise downloading onto your phone*

Downloading data takes power. Every time you download data onto your phone, it causes high levels of radiation to be emitted.

What are some of the main types of data that are downloaded onto phones? Emails, photos, videos, music and MMS (multimedia messages).

They are all data, yet they can vary enormously in size. As an example, a video clip will be far larger than a simple written email, and so will use more power.

Downloading big chunks of information causes the phone to emit far more power and radiation than it does when making a phone call.

> ". . . 207 billion MMS messages were sent in 2011."
>
> "In 2016, 387.5 billion MMS will be sent."
>
> **mobiThinking "Global Mobile Statistics"** *(2012)* **(32)**

Whenever you can, wait till you return to your home, office, or school computer before you attempt to download any material. If you can't wait, then make sure the phone is well away from you.

CELL PHONES - SAFETY TIP # 20

20. *Minimise web browsing and using apps*

Browsing the web and using apps to access information takes far more power than making a phone call.

The longer you spend connected to the Internet, the more power your phone uses, the more radiation it emits, the higher your exposure levels become. Preferably, wait until you're in front of a computer to connect to the net.

Unsurprisingly, app downloads are increasing exponentially. In 2010 the available apps were downloaded 10.9 billion times. In 2014, total downloads are predicted to reach 76.9 billion.

Once again, this is particularly important information for parents.

Because they have no idea of the consequences, young children are often given phones or tablets to play with, so that they can use apps as a distraction or entertainment.

> *"According to the Cellular Telecommunications and Internet Association, Americans spent a total of 2.2 trillion minutes on their mobile phones in 2008 - up 100 billion minutes from the previous year.*
>
> *Usage is expected to continue to rise, along with the use of other wireless devices and networks."*
>
> **Michael Lerner** *(2009)* *(33)*

CELL PHONES - SAFETY TIP # 21

21. Avoid listening to music on a phone

We've seen how your phone emits extra radiation whilst it's downloading music. Research is also telling us that phones can even affect us when they're in 'standby' mode.

For all the reasons given before, if you listen to music on your phone, you're also exposing yourself to far more radiation than if you were listening to music that's been stored on a standard Mp3 (preferably a non-wireless one).

CELL PHONES - SAFETY TIP # 22

22. Avoid passive radiation from phones

Like passive smoking, the effects of mobile phone radiation aren't limited to just the person using the phone. Passive radiation is being emitted from these phones - second-hand radiation that envelops everyone around the person while the phone is in use.

To help protect other people, keep at least three to six feet (1-2 m) away from them when you're using your phone - especially babies, children, and pregnant women – preferably more.

To protect yourself, keep the same distance from others when they're using theirs.

> "We all wish we'd heeded the early warnings about cigarettes. We think cell phones are similar."
>
> **Olga Naidenko** (2009) **(34)**

23. *Avoid the most intense radiation by keeping a distance away from phones*

As we've seen, the field of the most intense radiation around a phone extends directly around the phone in a sphere.

Whether you're texting, using the phone with an earpiece or loudspeaker, or carrying it in a bag, try to keep it at least a couple of feet (approx. 60 cm) away from you.

The further away from phones you are, the more the risks are minimised.

1. When you can, put the phone in a bag rather than carrying it in your hand.

2. When you're in a car, put the phone away from you in the passenger seat, rather than resting it in your lap.

3. When you're at home or at work, place it away from you on the desk, or the other side of the room if you can.

"Because mobile phones and other wireless gadgets are held close to the body and are used frequently, these devices are potentially the most dangerous sources of electromagnetic radiation that the average person possesses."

Olle Johansson *(2009)* *(35)*

---

24.   Keep the antenna away from you

The antenna is the main source of radiation from your phone.

In older models, the antenna used to be visible, but in most standard phones today it is usually hidden in the *top*. Many people mistakenly hold the *mouthpiece* away from them. This won't help. You need to keep the *antenna* away, especially from your head.

In some smartphones the antenna has been incorporated into the exterior or rim of the phone, making it harder to avoid.

If your fingers make contact with this, then the radiation will be conducted straight into your body. (One of the signs that this may be happening is reduced connectivity. The radiation is going into *you* instead of facilitating the connection.)

"What we have now are about 15 years of data that show that when you have the cell phone antenna close to your body, close to your head, close to your brain tissue - that it causes

➢   *a disruption in DNA repair, which is genetic damage.*

➢   *It causes leakage in the blood brain barrier, which is a special type of membrane in the blood vessels in your brain to protect brain tissue from toxic substances that circulate in your blood.*

And we now have about 14 epidemiological studies, studies of people who use cell phones, and the majority of those studies of people who use cell phones indicate an increase in the risk of developing both benign and malignant tumours."

George Carlo *(2005)* **(36)**

---

25. *Turn your Bluetooth capability off*

Just this one simple action can significantly reduce your exposure to radiation from not only your phone, but others' as well.

One thing you really should know about Bluetooth: all Bluetooth-capable devices within range (about 10 metres) automatically enter into a 'conversation' with each other, and they then form a 'personal area network'.

If one Bluetooth phone responds to a call, every other Bluetooth phone around will also react and try to transmit to the device, meaning that there is extra radiation emitted by all of them, filling the surrounded area with elevated levels of microwave radiation.

Turning the Bluetooth capability to 'Off' will stop your phone from responding to other phones and devices. This is especially important at night, when you're trying to sleep.

"... *We are constantly being bathed in an increasing sea of radiation from exposure to the above, as well as*

- *electrical appliances,*
- *computers,*
- *Bluetooth devices,*
- *Wi-Fi installations, and*
- *over 2,000 communications satellites in outer space that shower us with signals to GPS receivers.*"

Paul J Rosch (37)

---

26. Be aware that not all phones are equal
Simpler = Safer

Smartphones, superphones, Androids, BlackBerries, and PDAs can emit far more radiation than simpler standard phones because they are able to download large chunks of data.

This downloading of data uses high levels of power and increases radiation exposure. But more than this, it is the data being carried on the radio waves that is believed to be particularly harmful to health.

It's important to know this because if you're using this type of phone, you are potentially receiving more radiation than you would from a simple phone. As smartphones and superphones have become increasingly popular, this information has become relevant to more and more people.

The simpler and less sophisticated your phone - and the less capacity it has to download large chunks of data - the less radiation it will emit, the safer it is likely to be.

"Epidemiological studies show significant increased risk of benign and malignant brain tumors, acoustic neuroma, and melanoma of the eye and salivary gland tumors after ten years of cell phone use. Some studies suggest that even short-term use statistically increases cancer risk.

Neurological disease and autism have also been linked to wireless radiation exposure."

George Carlo *(2008)* *(38)*

---

27. Choose a 'low SAR' phone

Low SAR phones can help to reduce your overall exposure to radiation. (SAR stands for 'Specific Absorption Rate'.) When a phone has a low SAR rating, it means that the phone has lower emissions, and in theory you'll be exposed to less radiation.

However, while it helps, a low SAR rating for your phone is not a magic remedy. There are three things you should know about them.

➢ SAR ratings are an indicator only of how much thermal radiation is emitted by the phone, and how much will therefore be absorbed by your brain.

➢ That won't tell you anything about the non-thermal emissions that are now being connected with a variety of health issues.

➢ SAR ratings only apply when the phone is in a full signal area and are redundant when you're downloading any data, or websurfing.

"No cell phones are 'safe' - even if the SAR output is minimal. It's like the diet drink company telling you zero calories means 'healthy.'

I, and others, are concerned that this effort will actually be damaging to our question of fighting the implementation - because the focus will be on SAR, or calories - and not on whether the product is really healthy."

Vicki Warren *(2010)* *(39)*

You can find out the SAR rating of many phone models on:
"CNET: Cell phone radiation levels", and "EWG: Best and Worst Phones"

(There's more info on SAR in Hold The Phone: Here's Why pages 103-106.)

28. Beware trends and fashion marketing

It's important to remember that a mobile phone is not a fashion accessory or talking point. The bald truth is that it is a handheld radiation-emitting device. It exposes you to microwave radiation.

Mobile phone manufacturers and marketers are in business. They are not there to look after your wellbeing - they are there to make money.

One way of making sure that you keep sending your money their way is by linking phones to fashion trends. As long as you fall into line by buying multiple phones, or at least updating to the latest model, they know you'll play your part in the money chain.

However you choose to spend your money is your concern - as long as you're also aware of one important fact. Generally speaking, each new generation of phones features increased capability, and with that comes a potential increase in radiation exposure.

If you dare, flaunt your individuality, avoid following the pack and keep your old phone for as long as possible.

> *"It is not a good thing to proceed toward a world of ubiquitous wireless communication in a totally uncontrolled fashion."*
>
> **Ross Adey** *(2000)* **(40)**

29. To get a good night's sleep
Avoid making calls late in the day

Research has shown us that there is a direct link between exposure to electromagnetic radiation in general - and microwave radiation in particular - and disrupted sleep, shortened sleep, impaired quality of sleep, and also insomnia.

The timing is also interesting: As we continue to increase the amount of radiation in our air, more and more people complain of not being able to sleep properly.

According to *Sleep America* in the US, there has been a significant increase in sleeping problems since 2001.

➤ In 2001 the number of people getting eight+ hours sleep a night was 38%
  In 2009, it was down to 28%

➤ In 2001 13% people slept less than six hours a night on average.
  In 2009 that increased significantly to 20% - one in 5 people.

➤ In 2001 51% reported problems sleeping problems at least a few nights a week
  In 2009 that figure rose to 64% - **two out of every three people**

➤ 43% say they rarely or never get a good night's sleep on weeknights.

➤ 95% say they use some type of electronics, such as cell phones, within the hour before bed.

It seems more than possible that there's a direct link between the rate at which we are increasing our output of RFR, and the increased incidence of insomnia.

> *"The ones who were exposed reported headaches, it took longer for them to fall asleep and they did not sleep as well through the night . . .*
>
> *"If you have trouble sleeping, you should think about not talking on a mobile phone right before you go to bed."*
>
> **Bengt Arnetz** *(2008)* *(41)*

Babies and children are particularly vulnerable to external influences impacting on their sleep; and as many of us know, sleepless children almost always lead to sleepless parents.

Nearly *half* of all Americans have problems sleeping every night

and *two thirds* have problems sleeping some nights of the week.

Mobile Phone Radiation Wrecks Your Sleep

**Phone makers' own scientists
discover that bedtime use can lead to
headaches, confusion and depression**

"Radiation from mobile phones delays and reduces sleep, and causes headaches and confusion, according to a new study.

The research, sponsored by the mobile phone companies themselves, shows that using the handsets before bed causes people to take longer to reach the deeper stages of sleep and to spend less time in them, interfering with the body's ability to repair damage suffered during the day.

The findings are especially alarming for children and teenagers, most of whom - surveys suggest - use their phones late at night and who especially need sleep.

Their failure to get enough can lead to mood and personality changes, ADHD-like symptoms, depression, lack of concentration and poor academic performance.

The study - carried out by scientists from the blue-chip Karolinska Institute and Uppsala University in Sweden and from Wayne State University in Michigan, USA - is thought to be the most comprehensive of its kind."

The Independent, *January 20, 2008* **(42)**

Cell Phones - Safety Tip # 30

30. To get a good night's sleep - Cut down on the number of calls you make

Getting a good night's sleep is vital to your health. It's during deep sleep that your body is able to produce melatonin – which is a cornerstone of your immune function and hormonal system, and helps to maintain circadian rhythm,

There is a direct link between poor quality sleep, reduced melatonin levels, impaired immune function, reduced emotional wellbeing, and a variety of health conditions up to and including cancer. Even to weight gain. (Is this yet another way in which we are contributing to our rising obesity rates?)

> "The prominent influence of the circadian clock on human physiology is demonstrated by the temporal activity of a plethora of systems, such as sleep-wake cycles, feeding behavior, metabolism, physiological and endocrine activity, and even the rhythmic function of the heart, the brain and every single cell of a living body.
>
> Disrupted circadian rhythms will lead to attenuated feeding rhythms, unwellness, disrupted metabolism, and eventually to disrupted health."
>
> **Dimitris Panagopoulos** (2013) **(43)**

The microwave radiation that emanates from mobile phones - whether they're used for making calls, accessing the web, or downloading - is directly linked through research to reduced quantity and quality of sleep.

Exposure to microwave and electromagnetic radiation is known to impair melatonin production, which leads to disruption of the circadian 'clock'.

The more you use your phone, the more radiation you're exposed to (especially towards the end of the day), the more you risk your sleep being affected.

CELL PHONES - SAFETY TIP # 31

31. To get a good night's sleep -
Keep your phone away from you

Being near your mobile phone can disrupt not only how *much* you sleep, but also how *well* you sleep. In addition - the radiation from your phone can disrupt not only your sleep but also your production of melatonin, which goes on to affect your whole state of wellbeing.

This is really important, as so many people sleep with their phones right next to them. Many have their mobile on their bedside table and use it as an alarm clock.

Some children and teenagers even sleep holding onto their phones, or put them under the pillow so that they don't miss out on any contact with their friends during the night.

Disable your phone's capacity to transmit by switching it into 'airplane mode' and turning Bluetooth 'off' – and then keep it on the other side of the room.

> "When cells of the brain and nervous system leak, free calcium ions can enter the neurons from outside.
>
> Unscheduled steady calcium inflow due to electromagnetic radiation makes them more likely to release neurotransmitters, some of which will send false messages.
>
> This in turn can trigger brain hyperactivity leading, amongst other things, to sleep disturbances, loss of concentration (giving rise to ADHD) and stress headaches."
>
> **Andrew Goldsworthy** (2009) **(45)**

CELL PHONES - SAFETY TIP # 32

32. *Especially - when it's recharging*

The plug of mobile phone rechargers typically includes a transformer. Transformers often emit strong *magnetic* fields, which are high levels of low-frequency electromagnetic radiation. If your phone is on and recharging, you're then exposed to a *double* layer of radiation: microwave radiation coming from your phone, *and* magnetic fields from its recharger.

Make sure that your phone and recharger are either in another room, or on the other side of the room from you - especially while you're sleeping. If you have a couple of phones, and your partner does too, your bedside tables can start to resemble the flight deck in an airplane.For a good night's sleep, do what you can to keep your bedroom, and especially your bedside tables, free of technology.

> "According to a 2011 study of more than 3,500 people from 1,100 large corporations worldwide, 61 percent of those surveyed keep their cell phone in the bedroom, and more than four in ten have it within arm's reach while they sleep."
>
> **Larry Rosen** (2012) **(46)**

CELL PHONES - SAFETY TIP # 33

33.   Be cautious about using protection devices

Why the caution around products that are designed to protect you from the radiation coming from your phone? Because some of them don't work. And some of them may end up making you feel worse.

There are a variety of these on the market. They usually either claim to:

➢   *reduce* the amount of radiation that you're exposed to,

➢   *protect* you from the radiation that is being emitted, or

➢   *harmonize* the effects of the radiation.

Some you put on your phone, others you carry with you or wear. These are usually called personal protection devices.

A word or two of warning: At the time of writing it's very hard to substantiate any claims that these products will protect you from the effects of exposure to radiation. It's possible that some *may* help, but some definitely don't.

Protection devices that do work will potentially play a large part in the minimisation of our exposure one day. New devices are being worked on, but at the moment it's difficult to recommend current ones with any degree of confidence. However, as with all research in this field, things are constantly evolving. Keep you eyes open, and watch for new developments in this area.

Some people can feel better when they start using the devices. Many have seen their symptoms alleviated, only to watch them return over time. Sometimes this has happened after only a few weeks; for others it's taken months.

Unfortunately, some have experienced returning symptoms that were far worse than before they started using the devices.

Why do people stop feeling better? It's believed that this is due to the fact that even though a protection mechanism has been introduced, *the exposure has continued*. The cause - the source of radiation - hasn't been removed. This continual exposure leads to degeneration of health.

The symptoms that would normally indicate that this degeneration is happening are masked by the devices. In short, the damage is still occurring; but the early warning system has been disabled.

Over time, the damage increases until symptoms are again felt. By then, because the damage is worse, sometimes so are the symptoms.

This is such an issue that Dr George Carlo's *Safe Wireless Initiative* issued a general warning on the subject, which is available on: *www.etudesetvie.be/files/images/EMR-IP/Medicalalert-En.pdf*

"An alarmingly high number of patients with electro-hypersensitivity, and other related conditions, are reporting serious symptom relapses after periods of time when symptoms were apparently mitigated by use of products that claim to be protective against electro-magnetic radiation (EMR) related disease.

Several patients . . . are reporting symptom relapses that are believed to be more severe than the symptoms that led to their original diagnosis."

Safe Wireless Initiative (2008) *(47)*

There are two main reasons that protection devices are considered a problem.

1. **Due to the false sense of security they generate.** Some people feel that, as long as they have their device, they're protected. Instead of minimizing their use of phones, they keep on using them as much as they ever did; sometimes more.

The end result? Their levels of accumulated radiation exposure continue to rise until eventually their health may start to erode.

2.   **They can create more radiation**. Some accessories that are designed to reduce the radiation can actually reduce the connection quality.

As we've seen earlier, a reduced connection or signal results in the phone being forced to transmit at higher power. The end result: radiation levels actually *increase*.

Be cautious about using radiation protection devices either on your phone or yourself.

➢   If you do choose to use them, then be sure to research your chosen product very well.

➢   Look at the research behind any claims. If there are any studies, do their results match the marketing.

➢   Be aware that your phone will still be radiating and so you'll still be exposed. Continue to reduce your exposure by minimising your phone use.

➢   Limit their use. Use them only when you have to so that you don't override or disable your body's own protective capacity.

34. Keep cell phones for 'have to' calls only

While mobile phones emit microwave radiation, **corded** landline phones do not.

Each time you make a call on a landline phone, where the handset is connected to the phone via a cord, you're reducing your exposure to microwave radiation.

> *"Our results show that microwaves can cause irreparable damage. Our advice to people with mobile phones is not to use them if they have the option of using a land line."*
>
> **Levi Schachter** (2005) **(48)**

As your exposure to radiation is believed to be cumulative, every little counts.

Whenever you can, put your mobile to one side and make your calls on a **corded** *landline.*

> *"It is not generally appreciated that there is a cumulative effect and that talking on a cell phone for just an hour a day for ten years can add up to 10,000 watts of radiation.*
>
> *That's ten times more than from putting your head in a microwave oven."*
>
> **Paul J Rosch (49)**

35. Try to avoid becoming dependent on your phone

Research is showing us that there does appear to be a range of addictive behaviours displayed by many mobile phone users. They become especially distressed when separated from their phones (and/or computers).

"So 200 University of Maryland students agreed to go without social media for 24 hours - no cell phones or computers - and their reaction was akin to drug withdrawal.

Blogs written by students sounded desperate:

"In withdrawal. Frantically craving. Very anxious . . ."

"I am constantly on my phone. On average I probably send a text message every minute or so. I am ashamed that I couldn't go without my phone for 24 hours, but communicating with people is one of the most prominent things in my life."

"Texting and IM-ing my friends gives me a constant feeling of comfort," wrote one student. *"When I did not have those two luxuries, I felt quite alone and secluded from my life."*

The Washington Post, *April, 28, 2010* **(50)**

"The Nielsen Research Company found that during the final quarter of 2010 teens sent and received 3,705 texts each per month, which equals approximately six per hour."

Larry Rosen *(2012)* **(51)**

36.   When it's not in use, turn your phone off

Depending upon the model of your phone, most signal transmission capability is disabled by either:

➤ switching to airplane mode, and

➤ disabling Bluetooth, or

➤ turning it 'off'

Even in 'airplane mode' with some devices you can also turn Bluetooth and Wi-Fi mode back on – so double-check that everything is off.

This is most effective way of avoiding exposure, so whenever you can, turn to 'off' or 'airplane'.

"A scientist who maintains that mobile phones are safe to use is either corrupt or seriously incompetent."

PSRAST *(52)*
Physicians and Scientists for Responsible Application of Science and Technology

---

37. Be aware that every little step you take does count

It's believed that your exposure to radiation is cumulative - it all adds up. So each little step you take to reduce your exposure *does* count. It will help reduce your overall exposure load, especially in the long term.

And it's long-term use that scientists are particularly concerned about. The longer phones are used, the more radiation the user absorbs into their body.

The more radiation that's absorbed into the body, the higher the cumulative amount of radiation becomes: stepping ever closer to chronic exposure levels.

Research is showing us that chronic, long-term exposure levels are linked to a very wide range of health complaints - up to and including several cancers.

Studies link ten years phone use and over with increased risk of brain tumours.

"Studies led by Professor Lennart Hardell in Sweden found significantly increased risk of brain tumors from 10 or more years of cell phone or cordless phone use. Among their many significant findings are the following:

➤ For every 100 hours of cell phone use, the risk of brain cancer increases by 5%.

➤ For every year of cell phone use, the risk of brain cancer increases by 8%.

➤ After 10 or more years of digital cell phone use, there was a 280% increased risk of brain cancer.

➤ For digital cell phone users who were teenagers or younger when they first starting using a cell phone, there was a 420% increased risk of brain cancer."

L Lloyd Morgan (2009) *(53)*

"Cell Studies independent of industry funding show what would be expected if wireless phones cause brain tumors.

We would expect:
➤ The higher the cumulative hours of wireless phone use, the higher the risk
➤ The higher the number of years since first wireless phone use, the higher the risk;
➤ The higher the radiated power from cellphone use, the higher the risk;
➤ The higher the exposure (use on the same side of head as the brain tumor), the higher the risk] and;
➤ The younger the user, the higher the risk.

L Lloyd Morgan (2009) *(54)*

RECENT DISCOVERIES

Children and small adults absorb significantly more cell phone radiation than had been previously understood

"A new paper published online today in Electromagnetic Biology and Medicine demonstrates children and small adults absorb significantly more cell phone radiation than had been previously understood by using the conventional and widely used assessment methodology, the Specific Anthropomorphic Mannequin (i.e., plastic model of a brain, or SAM), to assess the "Specific Absorption Rate," known as the SAR.

Computer simulation of radiation penetration, in contrast to estimating radiation exposure using the fluid-filled plastic mannequin, demonstrates much greater radiation exposures, particularly for children and small adults, than previously understood.

The study shows that when phones are placed in the pocket or against the body the current FCC guidelines for radiation heating effects are presently being violated, and suggests that different SAR exposure guidelines should be established for people who are smaller than the mannequin, including children and smaller adults.

Experts say it is unlikely many cell phones on the market today would pass the FCC certification process with the amount of radiation now being demonstrated with this methodology."

Camilla Rees (October 2011) **(55)**

An Extract from the Warning by
Barrack Obama's 'President's Cancer Panel'

"Cell phone users can reduce their exposure to radiofrequency energy by:

➤ *making fewer calls,*

➤ *reducing the length of calls,*

➤ *sending text messages instead of calling,*

➤ *using cell phones only when landline phones are unavailable,*

➤ *using a wired "hands-free" device so that the phone need not be held against the head, and*

➤ *refraining from keeping an active phone clipped to the belt or in a pocket."*

"Unlike adults - even longer-term cell phone users - children have ahead of them a lifetime of RF and other radiation exposures and, therefore, special caution is prudent."

The President's Cancer Panel, April 2010 *(56)*

"...there is no absolutely safe level of exposure"

"Every cell phone must be connected to a base-station antenna to be functional.

Each connection results in a biologically active electromagnetic directional wave, which combines with the waves from other cell phones and wireless devices to form a mesh of information carrying radio waves (ICRW) from which there is little escape for most people.

The mechanism of harm perpetrated by ICRWs is biological and therefore carries no threshold for effects - in other words, there is no absolutely safe level of exposure.

All cells, tissues and organs in the range of exposure are therefore triggered, and the difference between people who develop symptoms and those who do not is related to factors such as age, state of wellness, gender and genetics."

George Carlo (2008) *(57)*

Cordless Phones

Quick Tips

Because it's not just mobile phones that cause concern

*"We do not err because truth is difficult to see.
We err because this is more comfortable."*

Aleksandr Solzhenitsyn

Cordless Phones at a Glance: The Issues

Just like mobile phones, cordless phones emit microwave radiation - but the radiation exposure from these can be *higher.*

What's the real issue with DECT phones?

Many people understand that there are health issues linked to using mobile phones, but very few realise that also includes *cordless* phones.

DECT (Digital Enhanced Cordless Telecommunications) phones pose real health issues, and there are two main reasons for that.

1. Firstly, the radiation that's emitted from the cordless **handset** when it's being used will penetrate your brain and body.

2. Secondly, the radiation that's emitted from the cordless **base station** will *fill your home with microwave radiation.* That causes a constant, twenty-four-hour exposure; not only for everyone living within that home, but often for those in many neighbouring homes as well.

***You're exposed to the radiation that's pouring out of the handset** and from the base station.*

➢ The more *powerful* the DECT phone, the more radiation that's being emitted - the higher the exposure for everyone in the home.

➢ The greater the *reach* of the phone, the more radiation that's being emitted - the higher the exposure for everyone in the home.

➢ The further away from the DECT base station you walk whilst making a call, the harder it has to work = more radiation and higher exposure levels.

Some cordless phone base stations in homes have been measured to emit more radiation than a mobile phone antenna on the street.

> *"Forget the health scares over mobile phones - the real danger could be the cordless landline in your home.*
>
> *New research shows the base stations of some cordless phones emit twice as much radiation as a mobile phone mast.*
>
> *Unlike mobile phones, the base stations put out radiation even when they are not in use, the study by Swedish scientists showed."*
>
> **Daily Mail Online**, February 6, 2006 **(58)**

Health Risks from Cordless Phones

Cordless phones use the same microwave radiation as mobile phones do. That means that the health risks and concerns are also the same.

Cordless phone use is linked with brain tumours. *Multiple* research studies provide evidence of this link.

> *"The evidence for risks from prolonged cell phone and cordless phone use is quite strong.*
>
> *For people who have used these devices for 10 years or longer, and when they are used mainly on one side of the head, the risk of malignant brain tumor is doubled for adults and is even higher for persons with first use before the age of 20 years ."*
>
> **Lennart Hardell** (2007) **(59)**

The Double Whammy

The radiation levels emitted from the handset when a call is being taken are far higher than the radiation emitted by the base stations of these phones. However, this does not mean that the radiation from the base stations is *safer.*

Why? Firstly, because we're discovering that there's most likely no such thing as any safe exposure level to microwave radiation.

And secondly, because it's a double whammy. Your exposure to the handset radiation is temporary (whilst you're making the call). Your exposure to the base station radiation is additional and permanent - it's on all the time.

Many DECT phones emit high levels of radiation 24/7. As so many people have them, it's the most common source of chronic radiation exposure in homes.

"A cordless phone of DECT standard is often the strongest source of high frequency electromagnetic radiation in a private home."

German Federal Agency for Radiation Protection *(2006)* **(60)**

"Is it really wise and safe to subject ourselves to whole-body irradiation, all around the clock and wherever we are, with the same mobile radiation which laboratory studies have shown to cause serious injuries and effects?"

Olle Johansson *(2009)* **(61)**

Non-Stop Pulsed 2.4 GHz Radiation Inside US Homes

Research Paper Abstract:

The use of DECT (Digital Enhanced Cordless Telecommunications) cordless phones has been a major health and environmental concern in Europe and especially in Germany for years . . .

The maximum power density was found to be over 500,000 µW/m2 at a normally encountered distance (about 1–2 feet), if the base station is placed on an office desk or bedside table.

The radiation peak values in the same room are higher than those encountered in proximity to cellular base stations located near residential buildings."

Haumann T and Sierk P (2002) *(62)*

Research Study: Haumann T, Sierk P. Non-Stop Pulsed 2.4 GH Radiation Inside US Homes

If you make only *one* change -
Replace your cordless phone with a *corded* handset

It's a simple but very powerful way to save your health.

Cordless Phone Safety Tips

What to do then?

How to protect your health?

*As well as the things we've already learnt
about mobile phones, the following are important
to know about cordless phones.*

*"Every truth passes through three stages before it is recognized.
In the first it is ridiculed.
In the second it is opposed.
In the third it is regarded as self-evident."*

Arthur Schopenhauer

CORDLESS PHONES - SAFETY TIP #1

1.   *The absolute priority - Change to a phone*

Because the base station of your cordless phone is emitting radiation all the time, it's constantly filling your home - the space in which you live, eat, sleep, and breathe - with microwave radiation.

The closer you are to the base station, the more radiation you're exposed to.

Because they emit radiation 24/7, DECT cordless phones are the biggest source of radiation exposure in many homes. Just being around cordless phones has the potential to cause a variety of health problems.

> *"There should be a clear distinction between a short-term exposure, like from speaking on a mobile phone close to the head, and long-term exposure from mobile phone base stations or DECT base stations."*
>
> **Gerd Oberfeld** *(2009)* **(63)**

Owning a cordless phone is just like putting a mobile phone tower right inside your own home. In contrast corded phones on landlines don't use microwave radiation.

By replacing your DECT cordless phone with a corded handset you're improving your potential for good health. Instantly. The second you take the plug out of the socket.

There is one thing to check here. The majority of landlines are connected via cabling in your home to the main phone lines in the street. With some new homes – particularly new apartment blocks – this is no longer the case.

Sometimes the cabled connections to the street phone lines are being replaced with wireless connections. Unfortunately, in terms of your radiation exposure, even if you're using a corded handset it still won't keep your home completely radiation-free.

If one of the reasons you're reluctant to give up your cordless phone is because you like to move around while you're making a call, then get a long extension lead so that you can walk around with the corded phone.

It may not be your dream solution, but it could keep you healthy.

"Many homes no longer have landline telephones, but only mobile or digital cordless (DECT) phones, which use the same technology as mobile phones.

If you have one, you have effectively installed the equivalent of a small mobile phone mast right inside your home or office."

Alasdair and Jean Philips *(2006)* ***(64)***

2. If you can't replace your cordless phone, use a 'low-radiation' cordless phone

Low-radiation phones can significantly help to cut down on your total radiation exposure.

Radiation will still be emitted from the handset but - as long as you're standing close to the base station - it will be less than from a standard cordless.

Radiation will still be emitted from the base station. But the most significant feature is that this will only happen *when it's in use* - while calls are actually being made.

The rest of the time the base station will not be radiating (or at least radiating at dramatically reduced levels) - meaning that you are saved from the majority of the radiation you're normally exposed to with a cordless phone.

"If you have a DECT with a base station in your house then you are filling your home with pulsing microwaves."

Alasdair Philips *(2006)* **(65)**

Cordless Phones - Safety Tip # 3

3. Keep the base station well away from areas in which people spend lots of time

As we've seen, microwave radiation is constantly pouring out of the cordless phone base station. It's this long-term, chronic exposure that's of particular concern when it comes to health.

Keeping away from the base station reduces your radiation exposure levels.

The closer you are to the base station, the more powerful the radiation, the higher your cumulative exposure levels, the more likely it is to affect your health.

"There is a body of evidence that warrants medical practitioners to take a precautionary approach to DECT technology and to, at the very least, advise patients with sleep and fatigue symptoms to avoid the use of DECT phones altogether.

The traditional wired phone may be more inconvenient, but may prove to be far safer in the long run.

If patients insist on having a DECT phone, at least advise them not to place the base station by the bed or anywhere where they spend extended amounts of time.

Don Maisch *(2006)* **(66)**

---

4. It's especially important to keep the cordless phone away from:

a your bedroom

Your body rests and repairs at night. Sleeping in a cloud of radiation can prevent that from happening. It can also stop you getting good quality sleep - or any sleep at all.

b a child's room

As we know, children are particularly vulnerable.

c anyone who's pregnant

It's not only young children that we have to be concerned about, but our *unborn* children too. It's particularly important to keep these as-yet-unformed children in an atmosphere that best allows them to develop to their full potential. Sleeping in a radiation-free environment is a very important part of that process.

d anyone who doesn't sleep well

It's *very* common to find that sleep can be disrupted by the radiation emitting from these cordless phone base stations. There are many anecdotal cases where people have been able to sleep again simply by turning the phone off. If someone is not sleeping well, the first thing you should consider is turning off the cordless phone at night.

e anyone who's already not well

If their immune system is already impaired, they need to be kept in a radiation-free environment, especially at night, to allow them the best chance of recovery back to full health.

5.   At the very least,
   Turn it off at night when you sleep

Just being around a DECT phone is well known to cause headaches and insomnia in some people (as well as a range of other health concerns).

The radiation only comes from the base station when it's turned on. If you can't replace your DECT phone, then turn it off whenever you're not using it. At the very least, turn it off at night.

Make sure to turn it off at the plug - or if there's no switch there, then unplug it completely to make sure there's no power coming through.

"The radiation exposure from a wi-fi router at 5 meters' distance, a cordless DECT phone base unit at 3 meters' distance, or digital baby monitor at less than 1 meter are all experienced at roughly the same level as a mobile phone mast only 150 meters away.

If any of these are closer, for example if you sleep with a cordless phone next to the bed, it is equivalent in radiation terms to being only about 50 meters away from a mast."

Wired Child *(67)*

---

6. *Save your neighbourhood by using a corded phone*

The range of some DECT cordless phones is so extensive that their radiation also affects the neighbours.

Even if your home is surrounded by rolling lawns, some phone systems are so powerful that the radiation reaches across the garden, penetrates through doors and walls and extends right into the houses next door. Sometimes even past that. Repeaters can also be attached to the phone. These increase the range and distance covered even more. Some brands' technical specifications claim that this can be extended up to three hundred metres around the phone.

The newer and more powerful the digital cordless system, the more reach it offers you, the more neighbours you can be affecting. And this works both ways: If *they* have a DECT phone system, the likelihood is that it's affecting *your* home as well. This is particularly common in apartments and townhouses where next door's base station can be literally on the other side of the wall.

Not sleeping well but know that there's nothing in your home to keep you awake? Perhaps this is your answer.

If possible, talk to your neighbours about this. Show them the evidence, and give them the resources to do their own research.

> *"The message taken out of this work is that people should be very cautious when using mobile phones next to their body (especially next to their brain), whereas the wireless DECT should be located as far away as possible from places that people use to spend many hours a day, not to mention children of all ages."*
>
> **Lukas H Margaritis** *(2012)* **(68)**

CORDLESS PHONES - SAFETY TIPS
7–9

As with mobile phones, if you just have to make a call on a cordless phone, it's *especially* important to:

7.   *Keep the call as short as possible*

8.   *Use the loudspeaker function*

9.   *Keep the handset well away from your head*

We know that a DECT cordless phone emits radiation constantly. But when a call is taken, the levels of radiation escalate dramatically - from both the base station and the handset.

If you pick up the handset and put it next to your ear, the high levels of microwave radiation go straight into your head. *The handsets of some DECT cordless phones emit more radiation than mobile phones.*

10. Avoid holding a cordless phone to just one side of your head

Regularly changing the side on which you hold the phone helps to reduce the intensity of the radiation exposure. It helps to protect your brain.

It's been shown through research that there is an increased risk of cancer - brain tumours - if the cordless phone is held to the same side of the head all the time.

"The risk of brain tumor (high-grade malignant glioma) from cordless phone use is 220% higher (both sides of the head).

The risk from use of a cordless phone is 470% higher when used mostly on only one side of the head.

For use of cordless phones, the increased risk of acoustic neuroma is three-fold higher (310%) when the phone is mainly used on one side of the head."

The BioInitiative Report *(2007)* *(69)*

Wireless and Computers

Quick Tips

Because it's not just phones that radiate . . .

"There are two ways to be fooled:
One is to believe what isn't so;
the other is to refuse to believe what is so."

Soren Kierkegaard

'WIRELESS' AT A GLANCE: THE ISSUES

Like mobile and cordless phones, all wireless appliances use microwave radiation, and also *emit* microwave radiation.

As with cordless phones, having wireless in the home can affect how you sleep, how your brain works, whether you remember things, your moods and how you behave, how well your immune system functions, whether you're able to conceive or not, how well you feel, and whether you're energized or not.

And don't forget that children are especially vulnerable to radiation from wireless appliances.

Wireless appliances affect more than just the person using the device.

Routers and wireless appliances can emit high levels of radiation, filling not just the room they are in, but often the entire home, the garden, and many neighbouring homes as well.

"Do not believe the Government or the Health Protection Agency when they say mobile phones (and by implication Wi-Fi) are safe; they are not.

They can cause excruciating pain to some 'electrosensitive' individuals, they interfere with normal brain function and have been shown to shatter the DNA in living human cell cultures.

All of this can be found in peer-reviewed scientific journals but, until now, has not been in the public domain."

Andrew Goldsworthy *(2008) (70)*

How do wireless appliances work?

The attraction of wireless appliances is usually due to both aesthetics and convenience. There are no restricting or ugly wires, and appliances can be used or operated from anywhere in the home. But how does that happen?

Take laptops as an example. In order for you to be able to use your laptop in any room of your home, it has to be able to pick up a signal. Wireless enables your computer to do just that. Because the router sprays a 'fog' of microwave radiation throughout your home your computer can pick up the signals and connect to the Internet.

Because it's invisible, and *most* people can't feel this radiation, they're not even aware of the difference they've caused to their living environment by inviting wireless into their homes.

The microwave radiation used for wireless is the same type of radiation that's used to operate mobile and cordless phones. And so it carries with it the same health risks.

Wireless Internet connections, and any other wireless-operated appliances can all fill your home with microwave radiation. Each time you install one of these, you bring another 'layer' of radiation into your home.

(How to know if something is 'wireless'? Generally, if the appliances aren't connected by cords or cables, then they are without wire: wireless.)

Wireless may be easier on the eye and more convenient, but there is a price to pay. All that convenience can come at the cost of your health.

You may hear the argument that wireless emissions are "lower than cell phone standards."

Yes, the *measurements* involved are lower; however, the risks and health effects are not.

Cell phone standards are put in place to protect you from the *short-term* exposure caused by holding a phone to your head.

With wireless, it's on all the time - and you're exposed to it 24/7. The emissions may be less; but cumulatively your *exposure* becomes far, far more as it is constant, *chronic* exposure.

It's also worth knowing that there is no universal agreement on these cell phone standards, with some countries having 'safety' levels that are thousands of times higher than those adopted by other governments.

(See the chapter on 'Safety Standards' in 'Hold the Phone: Here's Why' *to learn more about this.)*

Many scientists believe there is **no** safe level of exposure to microwave radiation.

With more and more people switching from cabled Internet connections to wireless connectivity, this has become a very serious issue for anyone concerned about public health - and their own health.

> "Manufacturers of devices that operate with wireless features should be required to carry SAR level information and warning labels on the outside packaging (not hidden inside).
>
> Wireless devices that create elevated RF levels for the user should be required to warn the user of possible adverse effects on:
>
> ➤ memory and learning
> ➤ cognitive function
> ➤ sleep disruption and insomnia
> ➤ mood disorders
> ➤ balance
> ➤ headache
> ➤ fatigue
> ➤ ringing in the ears (tinnitus)
> ➤ immune function
>
> and other adverse symptoms of use."
>
> **The BioInitiative Report** *(2007)* **(72)**

So how big an issue is wireless? How many people does it affect? In the US alone . . .

> "As of June 2011, there were more wireless subscriber connections (327.6 million) than the population of the US and its territories (315.5 million) . . . which means that wireless penetration rate in the US is now 103.9%.
>
> From January 2011 to June 2011, wireless data traffic increased 111% to 341 billion megabytes."
>
> **CTIA - The Wireless Association**
> *Blog, October 11, 2011* **(73)**

> *"New Wi-Max transmitters on cell phone towers, that have a range of up to two square miles compared to Wi-Fi's 300 feet, will soon turn the core of North America into one huge electromagnetic hot spot."*
>
> **Paul J Rosch** (74)

And what can be done to minimise the risks?

> *"We have established treatment to make these symptoms regress, however this does not prevent a recurrence.*
>
> *Thus, there is the necessity of adding protective measures to this treatment: creation of 'white zones', notably in public establishments and in public transport.*
>
> *We must do as for smoking: forbid Wi-Fi in certain zones, as in libraries. We must forbid installation of relay antennas near nurseries and schools.*
>
> *These are urgent protective measures to be taken, but are unfortunately not being applied."*
>
> **Dominique Belpomme** (2011) *(75)*

RECENT DISCOVERIES

Scientists Urge Halt of Wireless Rollout and Call for New Safety Standards:

Warning Issued on Risks to Children and Pregnant Women

"Scientists who study radiofrequency radiation from wireless technologies have issued a scientific statement warning that exposures may be harming the development of children at levels now commonly found in the environment. . .

Pregnant women are cautioned to avoid using wireless devices themselves and distance themselves from other users."

"The combined effect of cell phones, cordless phones, cell towers, Wi-Fi, and wireless Internet place billions of people around the world at risk for cancer, neurological disease and reproductive and developmental impairments."

"We are already seeing increases in health problems such as cancer and neuro-behavioural impairments, even though these wireless technologies are fairly new in the last decades or so for the general public. This finding suggests that the exposures are already too high to protect people from health harm."

"Safety standards also ignore the developing fetus, and young children who are more affected."

*Karolinska Institute Press Release (Feb 2011) **(76)***

Wireless Safety Tips

What to do then?
How to protect your health

*As well as the things we've already learnt about using
mobile and cordless phones,
the following are important to know about
computers and wireless.*

"*A truth's initial commotion is directly proportional to how deeply
the lie was believed.
It wasn't the world being round that agitated people, but that the
world wasn't flat.
When a well-packaged web of lies has been sold gradually to the
masses over generations, the truth will seem utterly preposterous
and its speaker a raving lunatic.*"

Dresden James

WIRELESS - SAFETY TIP # 1

1.   Replace any 'wireless' with wired

Wireless appliances and routers emit radiation whenever they are on. In most cases they're left on 24/7, which means that they're radiating *all the time*.

Replacing your wireless appliances with wired or cabled models is the best way of reducing your exposure to radiation.

Libraries switch off Wi-Fi Internet

Four libraries in Paris have turned off their Wi-Fi Internet connections after staff claimed they were causing health problems.

The latest to shut down its wireless network is the wireless Sainte-Genevieve university library in the 5th arrondissement after a member of staff threatened to take early retirement on health grounds.

In his letter to his employers, the shop worker stated: "Over the last few months, and increasingly over the last few weeks, I have suffered strong symptoms associated with the Wi-Fi network. . .

Symptoms have included headaches, balance problems, general weakness, stress and sight problems."

France 24, June 4, 2008 (77)

> *"There are many credible anecdotal reports of unwellness and illness in the vicinityof wireless transmitters (wireless voice and data communication antennas) at lower levels.*

> ➤ *Effects include:*
> ➤ *Sleep disruption*
> ➤ *Impairmentof memory and concentration,*
> ➤ *Fatigue,*
> ➤ *Headache,*
> ➤ *Skin disorders,*
> ➤ *Visual symptoms (floaters),*
> ➤ *Nausea,*
> ➤ *Loss of appetite,*
> ➤ *Tinnitus, and*
> ➤ *Cardiac problems (racing heartbeat)."*

> ***The BioInitiative Report*** *(2007)* *(78)*

WIRELESS - SAFETY TIP # 2

2. *Use cabled Internet*

You'll know by now that if you're using Wi-Fi, or any other wirelessly enabled Internet, you're sitting within a fog of microwave radiation. Simply changing the way you access the Internet can help to improve your health.

The number one preference to get you out of that radiation-fog-filled atmosphere, and to protect your health, is to change to cabled Internet.

Additional advantages are that cabled Internet connections are usually quicker, more secure, and offer better connectivity.

If wireless is built into your laptop, there is usually a switch that you can use to disable the wireless function. Just switch it to 'off' to make sure you prevent the appliance from emitting any frequencies. It's important to do this, even if your laptop is connected via a cable, and also remember to disable the wireless function in 'network connections'.

No-one is suggesting you give up the Internet, just *change* the way you access it.

Avoiding wireless routers is one of the simplest ways to protect your health - both now and in the long term.

"The following quote from the notes to editors* is muddled and deeply misleading."

> *"There is no consistent evidence to date that exposure to RF signals from Wi-Fi and WLANs adversely affect the health of the general population."*

It is muddled because it confuses two completely separate issues.

1. Is there any evidence that Wi-Fi is harmful to health?
*The answer to this is **DEFINITELY YES**.*

2. Is the whole population affected?
*The answer to this is **SEEMINGLY NOT**."*

Andrew Goldsworthy (79)

*Commenting on the Press Release by the Health Protection Agency
(September 15, 2009) Entitled "Scientist probe laptops Wi-Fi Emissions"

3. Be aware that all wireless appliances could affect your health

Wireless no longer just applies to phones and computers. There are a whole host of other appliances that work wirelessly, and that can pose a threat to your health.

As we know, in order for something that's wireless to work, signals are transmitted between the appliance and the controls. This means the intervening space needs to be filled with microwave radiation. Some devices only use wireless for remote controls, and in these cases the signal is short-lived (a bit like texting).

The longer the device is transmitting, the higher the levels of radiation exposure. The devices that constantly monitor and transmit radiation are the most detrimental to health.

> "Radiofrequency radiation (RF) - the part of the electromagnetic spectrum used in all-things-wireless today - is a known immune system suppressor, among other things. RF is a form of energetic air pollution and we need to understand it as such."
>
> **B Blake Levitt** (80)

Following are just some of the appliances that can be wireless:

➢ home office equipment, such as printers, scanners, etc.

➢ entertainment games, especially those with handheld devices or paddles

➢ digital baby monitors

➢ alarm systems for fire, burglary, etc with continuous monitoring/motion sensors

➢ tablets, notebooks, and book reader devices, which also rely on wireless in order to download their info

- DVDs, TiVo, and other TV and cable movie systems
- music and speaker systems

> "WI-FI routers, DECT phones and other wireless devices like baby monitors produce radiofrequency emissions that will affect millions of people and babies in their homes, and should be halted until other, less harmful options are investigated."
>
> **Lukas Margaritis** *(2011)* **(81)**

While normal TV remotes are usually ok, if you're able to turn the volume down on one of the latest TV's simply by waving your hands in the air, take the time to question: How can that be?

With any new technology, if there are no wires or cables, it's most likely to be wireless. Learn to look behind the lure of marketing to find out how the technology works, and how it's going to affect your health. Stay well away from any wireless devices that need to be carried on you, or worn on your body – especially your head.

It's assumed that everyone nowadays *wants* wireless appliances, so chances are that the salespeople won't even mention it. It's also likely that they're unaware that there *are* any potential health risks. Get into the habit of checking whether a product is wireless before you buy it; and if that's the case, ask if there's a wired alternative.

> "There's no question computer literacy is important . . . But you don't need Wi-Fi to do that. There's no question Wi-Fi falls into the category of a possible human carcinogen."
>
> **L Lloyd Morgan** *(2011)* **(82)**

Exposure to microwave radiation is believed to be cumulative. Even though you may be told that the exposure from each of these is "minimal" or "below international standards"*, it all adds up. Every little step in the right direction does count.

> *"Wi-Fi are just being rolled out as great big white heat of technology.*
>
> *Industry rules in this area and the precautionary principle, and the safety of people who might benefit to some extent from the technology, are completely dismissed.*
>
> *It's just . . . it's Wild West country for the companies. They just put them where they want and say there's no evidence."*
>
> **Ian Gibson** *(2007)* *(83)*

(*See the International Standards section in 'Hold the Phone: Here's Why' to find out more about that spin.)

WIRELESS - SAFETY TIP # 4

4.   *Save your neighbourhood by using cables*

Using wireless devices affects not just everyone in your house, but potentially all your neighbours as well.

Some wireless systems are so powerful that the radiation emitted extends not only throughout your home but also through the homes around you, especially in apartments and townhouses.

Just like DECT cordless phones, even if you live on a large block of land, the radiation from your system can extend beyond your garden and creep through the other homes in the neighbourhood. The reverse is also true: theirs can cross into your home.

How can you tell if someone else's Wi-Fi is intruding into your space? Plug in your laptop. If it's signalling that it's picking up Wi-Fi signals, then you know you are too.

> *"Depending on the intervening materials, a 'vanilla' Wi-Fi can radiate more than 1,000 feet.*
>
> *Since I live in a high-density area, my system reaches perhaps 100 neighbours."*
>
> **Nicholas Negroponte (84)**

Imagine in your mind's eye what would happen if everyone in a neighbourhood used Wi-Fi to access the Internet. The clouds of radiation circling out from the wireless router of each house would all overlap each other - adding layers and layers and layers of extra radiation to everyone's existing body burden.

This is already starting to happen; and like overlapping lily pads in a frog pond, it has been termed the 'lily pad effect.'

> *"Because further down the street, beyond the reach of my system another neighbour has put in Wi-Fi. And another, and another. Think of a pond with one water lily, then two, then four, then many overlapping, with their stems reaching into the Internet.*
>
> *In the future, each Wi-Fi system will also act like a small router, relaying to its nearest neighbours."*
>
> **Nicholas Negroponte (85)**

Changing to cabled Internet access not only increases your likelihood of good health, it also benefits your neighbours. Having cabled Internet helps to protect the health of all those living close to you. Especially their children. Even their pets.

5.   Say no to 'powerline networking'

However tempting it may seem, resist the urge to 'powerline network'.

Under this system, the radiation that's used to connect networked devices together transfers data along *the existing electrical wiring* buried within the walls of your house or office.

In piggy-backing on your electricity supply, the radiation can be conducted right along the wiring so that it's carried throughout your house. However, it doesn't necessarily stay confined to the wiring: it can extend out into the adjoining rooms. By installing powerline networking, you can unknowingly, but comprehensively, fill your house with microwave radiation.

Again, it's not just your house that's affected. As we're all connected via the shared electrical grid, this 'dirty electricity' can travel along the wiring and powerlines into the homes around you.

This method of information transfer is not restricted to wireless computers. Other wireless devices, such as entertainment systems, are now using the same method.

WIRELESS - SAFETY TIP # 6

6.   Keep your laptop off your lap

Despite their name, laptop computers are best kept right away from your lap. There are two main reasons for this.

1.   Even if they're not connected to Wi-Fi, the underside of laptop computers can give off very high electromagnetic radiation in the form of magnetic fields.

When you rest a laptop on your lap, you can be absorbing large amounts of this radiation into your body, especially your groin.

2.   When   laptops   are   connected   to   Wi-Fi,   they   become   a radiation-emitting device of even greater proportions, as they are then transmitting microwave radiation as well. A double dose of radiation that no one wants in their lap.

As laptops are used and held over the groin, there is real concern that they affect the fertility of those using them.

"There have been several studies showing that mobile phone use reduces male fertility. . . The prolonged use of a Wi-Fi laptop computer on or near the lap could have even more serious consequences for male fertility.

Anyone who considers Wi-Fi to be safe should think again."

Andrew Goldsworthy (2009) **(86)**

"We have demonstrated that exposure to laptops decrease progressive motility and induce DNA fragmentation in human spermatozoa in vitro by a non-thermal effect.

We speculate that keeping the laptops (Wi-Fi mode) on the lap near the testes may result in decreased male fertility."

Avendano C et al (2010) **(87)**

Research study: Avendano C et al. Laptop Expositions affect motility and induce DNA fragmentation in Human spermatozoa in vitro by a non-thermal effect: A preliminary report

7. Planes, Trains, and Automobiles: Avoid connecting and downloading when you're in them

Just like cell phones, using a wireless computer inside a metal structure exposes you to heightened radiation levels because the metal structure traps the radiation, and so the radiation accumulates instead of being able to disperse.

It's the wireless connection - the extra radiation involved in browsing or downloading - that poses the most risks to health, not your computer.

If it's not connected to Wi-Fi or Bluetooth, using your computer or notebook to write, read, listen, watch, or access information that's already stored there is not the issue.

This is very relevant for those who travel a lot in trains or planes; particularly for people who work under these conditions, such as pilots and cabin crew.

"People who are chronically exposed to low-level wireless antenna emissions report symptoms such as problems in:

- *sleeping (insomnia),*
- *fatigue,*
- *headache,*
- *dizziness,*
- *grogginess,*
- *lack of concentration,*
- *memory problems,*
- *ringing in the ears (tinnitus),*
- *problems with balance and orientation,*
- *and difficulty in multi-tasking.*

The BioInitiative Report (2007) **(88)**

(Another compelling reason not to allow the use of cell phones and wireless computers in airplanes.)

WIRELESS - SAFETY TIP # 8

As with cordless phone base stations, the microwave radiation that sprays from wireless routers and devices can affect everyone around them. If you just have to have them, it's especially important to:

8.   *Keep the wireless router away from people*

Avoid having them in rooms where people spend a lot of time, particularly bedrooms. This is very important for anyone who is:

➤   young, or elderly
➤   pregnant
➤   unwell, or
➤   unable to sleep

This is, of course, also important for workplaces – where many spend their days and weeks in environments that are overflowing with radiation from a variety of sources.

Check out your office or workplace to see where routers and other devices are located. How close are they to you?

WIRELESS - SAFETY TIPS # 9-11

And, for the same reasons ...... it's also especially important to:

9.   *Turn the router off when you're not using it*

Any time the router is on, it's filling the room (or rooms) with radiation. If you have to use a router to access the Internet or download material, try to get into the habit of turning it on only when you need to, and then remember to turn it off again as soon as you're done.

10.   *Turn the wireless function off when you're not using it*

Ditto with wireless function. If you need to use the wireless function on laptops, tablets, readers, etc to download material, then make sure it's only on while you're actually downloading (and move away from it while that's happening). Remember to turn it off or into 'airplane mode' afterwards.

11. Make sure to turn it all off at night

There is little doubt that microwave radiation interferes with both the ability to get to sleep, and the quality of sleep. It also affects the production of melatonin, which is produced when we sleep and is the cornerstone of an effective immune system.

To get a good night's sleep, and to stay healthy, try to make sure that you're sleeping in as radiation-free an environment as you possibly can. Turn everything possible 'Off'.

"The study indicates that during laboratory exposure to 884 MHz wireless signals, components of sleep, believed to be important for recovery from daily wear and tear, are adversely affected."

Arnetz B et al (2007) **(91)**

Research study: Arnetz B et al. The Effects of 884 MHz GSM Wireless Communication Signals on Self-reported Symptom and Sleep (EEG)- An Experimental Provocation Study.

"Prolonged exposure to radiofrequency and microwave radiation from cell phones, cordless phones, cell towers, Wi-Fi and other technologies has been linked to:

➢ interference with short-term memory and concentration,

➢ sleep disruption,

➢ headaches and dizziness,

➢ fatigue,

➢ immune disruption,

➢ skin rashes, and

➢ changes in cardiac function"

Martin Blank (2007) **(92)**

Children and Phones

Quick Tips

"The truth is like the sun.
You can shut it out for a time, but it ain't goin' away."

Elvis Presley

Children: Why They Are a Special Case

"Our children are our only hope for the future,
but we are their only hope for their present and their future."
Zig Ziglar

Why so many warnings about children using mobile phones?

Because the radiation from mobile and cordless phones affects children far more than adults. In fact, because their brain is still developing, that's the case for anyone under twenty.

The *younger* they start using mobile phones, the *earlier* the physical effects of radiation exposure may begin to become apparent.

If a child starts using a phone at age 8, the ten-year latency period for phone-induced tumours could be reached by only 18.

Children are far more vulnerable than adults

There is a big difference between an adult using a mobile or cordless phone and a child using one. Children are far more vulnerable to the radiation that is emitted by them because:

➢ Their bone structure is thinner, and their skulls are less developed. This means that the radiation can enter into the brain *more easily*.

➢ They have smaller heads than adults, allowing proportionally *more* radiation to be absorbed.

➢ Because of all this, the radiation penetrates *more deeply* into children's brains. The younger the child, the more of their brain it 'fills'.

➤ It's believed that children's brains are *more conductive* than adults, allowing the radiation to circulate around the brain more rapidly.

➤ Children's brains are considered *more sensitive* and so are more likely to be affected by the radiation.

➤ A child's brain is still growing and forming. Radiation may endanger the development of the brain.

"When you start talking about a child 8 or 9 years old beginning [cell phone] use, by the time they are 18 or 19 years old, they will have used the phone for 10 years.

The projections that we do have indicate that we are putting these children in unbelievable danger."

George Carlo *(2009)* **(93)**

➤ A child's nervous system is still developing. Brain wave activity is more vulnerable to disruption by microwave radiation, particularly children with epilepsy, ADD, and ADHD.

➤ Children's alpha brain wave rhythms are not fully stabilized, meaning their cognitive function, creativity, and positive moods are more likely to be disrupted.

➤ A child's immune system is less developed. The concern is that consistent exposure to microwave radiation may hinder long-term immune function.

➤ Children are far more susceptible to genetic damage than adults. (Genetic damage can be a precursor to cancer.)

➤ Children are far more sensitive and vulnerable to all the effects of exposure to electromagnetic radiation.

➤ Children's cumulative exposure to radiation is far greater. The younger the children are when they start using mobile or cordless phones, the longer they will be exposed to the radiation.

This means that 'long-term exposure' can be reached by the time children become teenagers.

> "The results show that children's brains are affected for long periods even after very short-term use. Their brain wave patterns are abnormal and stay like that for a long period. This could affect their mood and ability to learn in the classroom if they have been using a phone during break time, for instance."
>
> These same altered brain waves "could lead to things like a lack of concentration, memory loss, inability to learn and aggressive behaviour."
>
> "If I were a parent I would now be extremely wary about allowing my children to use a mobile even for a very short period. My advice would be to avoid mobiles."
>
> **Gerald Hyland** (2001) **(94)**

The latest in research . . .

Double the radiation absorption in children

'. . . the electrical properties of tissues – especially of the head – in all animals change with age.

The relative permittivity* of an adult human brain is calculated to be around 40 while the corresponding value for a young child's brain is between 60 and 80 resulting in almost double the radiation absorption and SAR.'

Panagopoulos DJ, Johansson O, Carlo GL (2013) **(95)**

Research: Panagopoulos DJ, Johansson O, Carlo GL (2013) Evaluation of Specific Absorption Rate as a Dosimetric Quantity for Electromagnetic Fields Bioeffects

* the ability of a substance to store electrical energy

The age and size of the child makes a difference

The smaller and younger the child, the greater the penetration of the microwave radiation into their brain, as you can see from the illustration below:

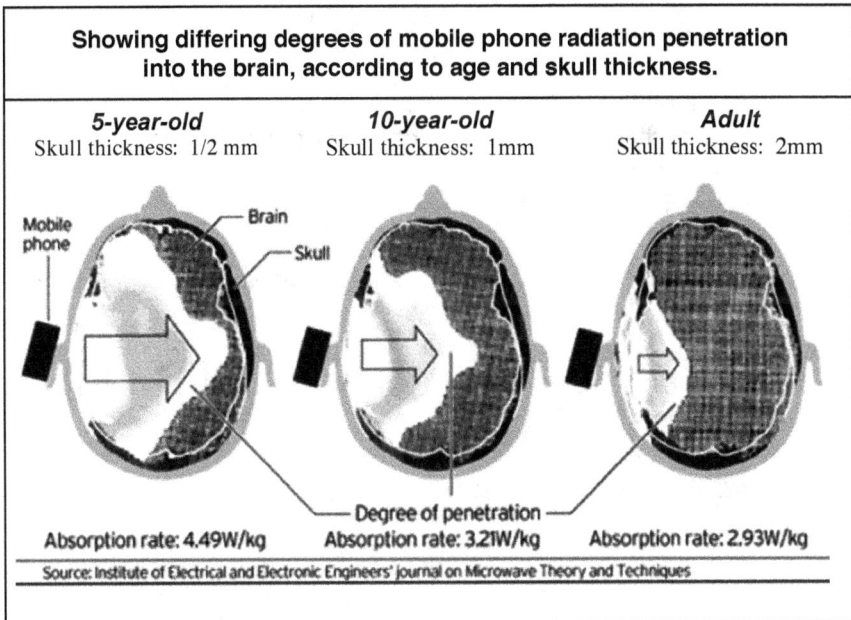

Showing differing degrees of mobile phone radiation penetration into the brain, according to age and skull thickness.

5-year-old	*10-year-old*	*Adult*
Skull thickness: 1/2 mm	Skull thickness: 1mm	Skull thickness: 2mm
Absorption rate: 4.49W/kg	Absorption rate: 3.21W/kg	Absorption rate: 2.93W/kg

Degree of penetration

Source: Institute of Electrical and Electronic Engineers' journal on Microwave Theory and Techniques

Energy deposition for models of an adult, and 10- and 5-year old children, for a cellular telephone at 835 MHz. Radiated power = 600 mW. (From O P Gandhi et al, IEE Trans. Microwave Theory & Techniques, 44, p 1893, 1996) Reproduced with the kind permission of Professor Om P Gandhi, University of Utah, USA.

"When electrical properties are considered, a child's head's absorption can be over two times greater, and absorption of the skull's bone marrow can be ten times greater than adults.. ."

Om P Gandhi *(2012)* **(96)**

Research study: Gandhi OP. Exposure limits: the underestimation of absorbed cell phone radiation, especially in children

All this is particularly concerning when you see the statistics on cell phone ownership - not use, just ownership - amongst our very young. According to research published by the Kaiser Family Foundation in the US in 2010, the percentage of those *owning* a cell phone in 2009 was:

➢ 31% of 8-10 year olds
➢ 69% of 11-14 year olds
➢ 85% of 15-18 year olds

Four years is a long time in the evolution of the cell phone market, and it's highly likely that those figures are a lot higher today. (Please note also that these figures do not take into account the number of children using cordless phones at home, which pose similar risks.)

In 2011 the GSMA published the following statistics on children's use of mobile phones:

Children's use of mobile phones - An international comparison 2011

➢ 70% of all children surveyed use a mobile phone.

➢ Children show higher smartphone use than their parents.

➢ Children send more messages as they get older, peaking at 15.

➢ 40% of children access Internet via mobiles; usage increases with age.

➢ 70% of children in Japan and Portugal who use mobile Internet, do so for more than 30 minutes a day.

➢ Primary Internet access for 56% of Japanese children is via smartphone

GSMA, NTT DOCOMO 2012 (2011) (97)

"Children who use cell phones have more than a five-fold (500%) increased risk of malignant brain tumor by the time they reach the 20–29 age-group."

Cindy Sage (2008)) (98)

In the short term, the most common health effects on children from this radiation are issues with:

- ➢ memory
- ➢ mood swings
- ➢ learning and cognitive function
- ➢ behaviour
- ➢ irritability and aggression

- ➢ sleep
- ➢ impaired development
- ➢ hyperactivity
- ➢ attention/concentration and ADD

The long-term effects are the same as for adults, except they can appear in children far more quickly, and whilst they are still very young.

"The following health hazards are likely to be faced by the children mobile phone users in the nearest future:

- ➢ *disruption of memory,*
- ➢ *decline of attention,*
- ➢ *diminishing learning and cognitive abilities,*
- ➢ *increased irritability,*
- ➢ *increase in sensitivity to the stress,*
- ➢ *sleep problems,*
- ➢ *increased epileptic readiness."*

Russian National Committee on Non-Ionizing Radiation Protection (RNCNIRP) *(2008)* **(99)**

(For more details, see the Symptoms section in the chapter on Health in 'Hold the Phone: Here's Why'.)

Autism Spectrum Disorder (ASD):

The latest figures on autism paint a sobering picture:

➢ One in 88 children is identified with an autism spectrum disorder.

➢ The 2012 CDC *(Centers for Disease Control and Prevention)* report states "about *1 in 6 children* in the U.S. had a developmental disability in 2006-2008, ranging from mild disabilities such as:

- speech and
- language impairments

to serious developmental disabilities, such as
- intellectual disabilities,
- cerebral palsy, and
- autism."

➢ Reported ASD rates in 1975: 1 in 5000.

➢ By 1995, it was 1 in 500.

➢ Autism rates continue to escalate. They *double* every five years.

"The percentage of children diagnosed with ADHD rose 33% from the late 90s to 2008, with 10 million children ages 3–17 diagnosed with a developmental disorder.

*In the past decade alone the percentage of children with ADHD rose an **additional** 30%."*

Larry Rosen *(2012)* **(100)**

According to the BioInitiative Report 2012, there are many similarities between the symptoms of ASD and the bioeffects of RFR exposure.

Among these similarities are:

➢ oxidative stress and free radical damage

➢ altered brainwave activity and altered nervous system

➢ electrophysiology

➢ sleep disruption

➢ immune system dysfunction

➢ possible blood brain barrier leakage

➢ poor mitochondrial function

➢ stress

And behavioural irregularities shared by both are:

➢ agitation and hyperactivity

➢ short attention span

➢ aggression

➢ unusual sleeping habits

➢ moods, or unusual emotional reactions

➢ in some cases, heightened fear and anxiety

Interestingly, these are also some of the characteristics of electrosensitivity *(see the 'Electrosensitivity' chapter in* 'Hold the Phone: Here's Why'.*)*

As you'll see over the following pages, research has also shown that in-utero exposure to cell phones resulted in offspring that were more likely to display behavioural traits similar to those of ASD.

Because children with ASD already display signs of neurological problems, it's particularly important that this is not aggravated. Providing them with living environments that are as free as possible of any electromagnetic radiation is an important step in this process.

Exposure to cell phones and wireless communications have been linked with Autism.

> *"The findings suggest a significant role of EMR in both the etiology of Autism and the efficacy of therapeutic interventions.*
>
> *These data also suggest that wireless device EMR is a synergen in the etiology of Autism, acting in conjunction with environmental and genetic factors, and offer a mechanistic explanation for the correlation between concurrent increases in the incidence of Autism and the use of wireless technology."*
>
> *Mariea T, Carlo GL* *(2007)* **(101)**
> *Research study: Mariea T, Carlo GL. Wireless Radiation in the Etiology and Treatment of Autism: Clinical Observations and Mechanisms*

It has been observed that some children with ASD have experienced some relief from symptoms when they are placed in environments that are either low-EMR or EMR-free.

The most important step in providing this cleaner, less agitating environment is eliminating wireless from the home, and ensuring that all phones, computers, and appliances are wired and corded.

Don't forget our unborn children

It's not only our children who are more vulnerable to environmental toxins, but also our unborn children.

One of the reasons that children's vulnerability is high is due to their rapid growth rate. Fetuses have an even faster rate of growth.

It appears that how, and to what extent, the development of the child is affected depends upon - among many other factors - which biological systems were developing at the time the fetus was exposed to radiation.

There are certain important 'windows of critical development' within the growth and development of the fetus during gestation. Exposure during these 'windows' appears to exacerbate the results. It's believed this may have, in some cases, potential to affect the long-term health of the child.

The levels of exposure are also relevant. Obviously, if the exposure to the fetus is consistent and chronic, then the risks to overall physical, neurological, mental, and emotional development are higher.

One 2012 study on mice showed that offspring who had been exposed while in-utero displayed behaviour that was similar to ADHD, and concluded this was due to impaired neuronal development (Aldad et al).

A 2009 study in Greece reported altered development of cranial bones of the fetus (Fragopoulou et al). This was from low-intensity exposure, yet further indication that bioeffects are not necessarily related to the strength/intensity of the exposure. It's more complex than that.

A giant study by Divan et al in 2008 found significant behavioural differences in children born to mothers who used mobile phones.

Because the vast majority of expectant couples have absolutely no idea of the possible effects to their future children, many make countless phone calls throughout the day, and their houses are bathed in a constant fog of radiation from DECT phones and wireless appliances (that are simply there because they offer enhanced convenience).

"Women who use mobile phones when pregnant are more likely to give birth to children with behavioural problems, according to authoritative research.

A giant study, which surveyed more than 13,000 children, found that using the handsets just two or three times a day was enough to raise the risk of their babies developing hyperactivity and difficulties with conduct, emotions and relationships by the time they reached school age.

And it adds that the likelihood is even greater if the children themselves used the phones before the age of seven. And when the children also later used the phones they were, overall, 80 percent more likely to suffer from difficulties with behaviour.

They were:

➢ *25 percent more at risk from emotional problems,*

➢ *34 percent more likely to suffer from difficulties relating to their peers,*

➢ *35 percent more likely to be hyperactive, and*

➢ *49 percent more prone to problems with conduct.*

Professor Sam Milham, of the blue-chip Mount Sinai School of Medicine in New York, and the University of Washington School of Public Health . . . pointed out that recent Canadian research on pregnant rats exposed to similar radiation had found structural changes in their offspring's brains."

The Independent, *May 18, 2008* **(102)**

This knowledge is vital for anyone wishing to have children so that they are aware of the importance of minimising their exposure to the radiation from cell phones, cordless phones, Wi-Fi, and other wireless appliances.

If possible - Start minimising your exposure before you fall pregnant.

There is adequate evidence today to suggest that those wishing to have families should do all they can to minimise their exposure to RFR radiation well *before* attempting to fall pregnant.

This seems to be particularly the case for men, where constant phone exposure has been shown to actually work contra conception. The radiation affects both the quantity and the quality of the sperm. This can impact on the likelihood of conception, and also the potential health of the child-to-be.

As mentioned in the chapter on cell phones, exposure to RFR has also been linked to increased incidence of miscarriage.

Because of our new wireless environment, it seems that recommend-ations for preconception care are now a good idea for *anyone* planning a family in the future.

To sum up, there is a two-stage exposure to unborn children:

1. Preconception radiation exposure that has occurred to both parents, affecting the testes/sperm of the father, and the ovaries of the mother - the genetic foundation for the unborn child.

2. In-utero radiation exposure while the child is still being carried by the mother: direct cell phone exposure; passive radiation from other phones nearby; and also the ambient exposure from DECT phones and other wireless appliances in the living and working environment of the mother.

Protecting the long-term health of children extends beyond the very young. As we've seen, it is best started pre-conception, is critical in-utero, and requires vigilance and consistency as they grow up. However, this care does not tail off until children reach their early twenties, as it is not until then that the maturation of their nervous system is said to be complete.

> *"Scientists at the Children with Cancer conference in London this week will advocate that governments adopt the 'precautionary principle' - advising phone users to take simple steps to protect themselves and their children from potential, not proven, long-term health risks of electromagnetic fields - especially head cancers.*
>
> *They will call for urgent research into new Office of National Statistics figures that suggest a 50 per cent increase in frontal and temporal lobe tumours - the areas of the brain most susceptible to the electromagnetic radiation emitted by mobile phones - between 1999 and 2009."*
>
> **The Independent**, *April 24, 2012*   *(103)*

There are always alternatives. It is possible to make phone calls using a corded handset on a landline. It is possible to connect to the Internet via wired computers. These are important personal choices that each potential parent needs to consider.

This level of radiation exposure is something that we as a race have never before experienced. We still have no idea of the full ramifications into the future.

Protecting our unborn children, our current youngsters, and our future generations has to become our most urgent priority.

While this is concerning information for those with children, it was felt necessary to include it – especially for the sake of future parents.

*If you are a parent, and you're now aware that your child has been exposed to this radiation, it's really important not to panic, or to go into guilt. (For many there's enough guilt involved in parenting anyway.) Please remember that this research is providing us with a link to potential effects, **not** a foregone conclusion that they will happen. We are all individuals, and it appears that not everyone is always affected. We all differ in the way we're affected, or not - and how much we're affected, or not.*

More information about the effects of children using mobile and cordless phones

The ICEMS (International Commission on Electromagnetic Safety) has recently announced a **Campaign for Safer Cell Phone Use,** aimed specifically at young children, teens, and pregnant women.

This information includes FAQs, videos, and links to other informative websites, and can be found at _www.icems.eu/public_education.htm._

Other good sources of information are the downloads available from both *Powerwatch* and *Mobile Wise*, details of which are given in the Articles, Letters and Reports section *(on pages 207-208).*

"Our recent 4-year monitoring of effects from cell phone radiation on children . . . demonstrates an increase in phonemic perception disorders, abatement of efficiency, reduced indicators for the arbitrary and semantic memory and increased fatigue.

Over the four-year monitoring of 196 children ages 7-12 who were users of mobile communication devices, a steady decline in these parameters from high values to bottom standards compared was observed.

The short-term and long-term potential consequences for society from exposing children to microwave radiation from cellular communication devices must be immediately acknowledged, globally, and responsibly addressed."

Yuri Grigoriev *(2011)* *(104)*

Mobile Phone use
'raises children's risk of brain cancer fivefold'

Professor Hardell told the conference that "people who started mobile phone use before the age of 20 had more than five-fold increase in glioma . . ."

The extra risk to young people of contracting the disease from using the cordless phone found in many homes was almost as great, at more than four times higher . . .

"This is a warning sign. It is very worrying. We should be taking precautions."

He believes that children under 12 should not use mobiles except in emergencies and that teenagers should use hands-free devices or headsets and concentrate on texting.

At 20 the danger diminishes because then the brain is fully developed."

The Independent; *September 21, 2008* **(105)**

"Controlling cell phone use in young people is not a choice. It is an urgent necessity."

George Carlo (106)

"If medications delivered the same test results as mobile phone radiation, one would have to immediately remove them from the market."

Erik Huber (107)

"In a world where a drug cannot be launched without proof that it is safe, where herbs and natural compounds available to all since early Egyptian times are now questioned, their safety subjected to the deepest scrutiny, where a new food cannot be launched without prior approval . . .

. . . the idea that we can put up mobile telephony masts and introduce Wi-Fi willy-nilly around our 5-year-olds is double-standards gone mad.

And I speak, not just as an editor and scientist that has looked in depth at all the research, but as a father that lost his beloved daughter to a brain tumour."

Chris Woollams *(108)*

Children's Safety Tips

What to do then?
How to protect their health

*"Children are one third of our population
and all of our future."*

Select Panel for the Promotion of Child Health (1981)

1. Children are more vulnerable. Keep them well away from mobile phones, cordless phones, and wireless

As we've seen, children are far more sensitive to radiation than adults.

The younger and smaller they are:

➢ the more vulnerable they are to microwave radiation,

➢ the more effect the radiation has on their biology.

> "Children are more severely affected (by radiation) because their brains are developing, and their skulls are thinner.
>
> **A two-minute call can alter brain function in a child for an hour**, which is why other countries ban their sale or discourage their use under the age of 18."
>
> **Paul J Rosch (109)**

Official advice from government bodies the world over is overwhelmingly to prevent children - and even teenagers - from using mobile phones, cordless phones, and wireless appliances. The best phones for children to use are **corded** landlines.

Their immune systems, their hormonal systems, and their brains are still growing and developing. Research is leading us to believe that exposure to microwave radiation at this tender stage of growth may be hindering their development and impacting on their chances of good physical and mental health in adulthood.

Have a look at the chapter on Official Warnings (in Hold The Phone: Here's Why) to see just how many governments have issued warnings about children's exposure to this radiation.

"A child's skull is not only thinner and surely has different dielectric properties because it has more blood vessels - it also contains many more stem cells which can form blood cells.

Hence, if RFMW radiation has an influence on the development of cancer, its effects will be greater for two reasons:

First, the most vulnerable cells are only millimetres from the antenna.

And second, the earlier in life a malign transformation occurs, the more likely it will result in a clinical malignancy."

Michael Kundi (2002) *(110)*

"And the concern is not just brain tumors, but other health effects associated or reported to be associated with cell phones, including behavioral disturbances, salivary gland tumors, male infertility and microwave sickness syndrome . . .

And with so many users and users starting at the age of three and up now, we should be concerned."

Vini Khurana (2008) *(111)*

"Since children's nervous systems are still developing, and they have thinner scalps and skulls than adults. They should use cell phones only in emergencies."

Gene Barnett *(112)*

CHILDREN - SAFETY TIP # 2

2.   *Text instead of talking*

A phone call results in sustained exposure - right next to the brain.

When a child sends, or receives a text, it doesn't involve them having to put the phone next to their ear.

Unlike calling, texting also results in a comparatively short burst of radiation - usually when the phone is held away from their head.

If your children are in a situation where they need to use a mobile to communicate, it's much better and safer for them to text than to talk.

"More radiation can go through since the child's ear is thinner, the telephone is closer to the head, and this thinner ear doesn't absorb so much power.

Therefore, more is able to go past the ear into the head. All it takes is two millimetres difference."

Om Gandhi (2001) (113)

---

3.   *Keep it brief*

If your child just has to talk on a mobile or cordless phone, remember to keep the call as brief as possible.

And keep changing the handset from ear to ear to dissipate the effect.

Mobile telephone use is associated with changes in cognitive function in young adolescents

➤   *"The accuracy of working memory was poorer,*
➤   *reaction time for a simple learning task shorter,*
➤   *associative learning response time shorter, and*
➤   *accuracy poorer*
in children reporting more mobile phone voice calls."

Abramson MJ et al *(2009)* **(114)**

Research study: Abramson MJ et al. Mobile telephone use is associated with changes in cognitive function in young adolescents

---

CHILDREN - SAFETY TIP # 4

4.   Mobile phones are not toys

Mobile phones are not like the simple corded phones we used to use. Nor are they toys or entertainment centres. They are, literally, handheld radiation-emitting devices.

Instead of being offered phones to play with as a distraction, children need to be protected from them.

Offer them corded or battery, non-wireless entertainment.

Discussing the 1 to 2% annual increase in childhood brain cancers

"It's not age, it's too fast to be genetic, and it isn't all down to lifestyle, so what in the environment can it be?

We now live in an electro-smog, and people are exposed to wireless devices that we have shown in the lab to have a biological impact.

It makes sense that kids are more sensitive - they have smaller heads and thinner skulls, so EMFs get into deeper, more important structures.

It is totally unethical that experimental studies are not being done very fast, in big numbers, by independently funded scientists."

Annie Sasco *(2012)* **(115)**

---

5. Be aware that wireless games systems emit radiation

The consoles of these entertainment, exercise, and gaming systems can give off fields of radiation large enough to fill a home. It's not just the consoles that are a concern - the remotes also emit radiation.

The instructions that accompany some consoles warn of the effect on cardiac pacemakers and other implanted medical devices. There is also a general warning given about exposure to radio frequency radiation, and recommendations to keep a distance between the consoles and anyone using them.

The consoles are also often left on all the time, even when they're not being played with - adding to the list of appliances that emit radiation around the clock.

It's safest to stick with entertainment systems and games that function via wires and cords.

"**Concern 7**: The danger of brain tumors from cellphone use is highest in children, and the younger a child is when he/she starts using a cellphone, the higher the risk.

Compounding this concern is a recently published Swedish study reporting a 420% increased risk of brain tumors from cellphone use, and a 340% increased risk from cordless phone use when wireless phone use began as teenagers or younger."

L Lloyd Morgan (2009) (116)

6. *Avoid using digital cordless baby monitors*

Most people understand the need for baby monitors. However, there are few who understand that there's an important difference between using wired or analogue baby monitors and using a (DECT) cordless model.

DECT cordless baby monitors use the same technology as cordless phones. Essentially, they fill the air with a fog of microwave radiation. (The older cordless baby monitors were analogue and didn't pose the same dangers to a baby's health.) If you're this far into the book you'll already understand the implications of this, especially for young babies, who are our most vulnerable group.

Fact for new parents: The latest cordless monitors use microwave radiation. Microwave radiation has been shown to interrupt sleep patterns. The last thing any parent of a newborn needs is an appliance that is going to prevent their baby from sleeping.

"Baby monitors are typically placed close to infants, who are particularly at risk from radiation . . .
Babies are especially vulnerable because their bodies and nervous systems are still developing and because they will have more time to accumulate exposure to the radiation and for any delayed effects to develop.

The Independent, May 20, 2007 (117)

"It is recommended that advice to new parents would be to have nothing to do with DECT baby monitors whatsoever."

Don Maisch (2006) (118)

"Over the past five years we, with the help of parents, have measured a variety of baby monitors and the DECT pulsing ones seem to be far more disruptive of the infant's sleep and state of contentment (causing restlessness, irritability and crying).

We have had a number of reports from parents that their babies did not sleep well and cried a lot when they used DECT monitors, but were ok when no baby monitor was used. When they then tried a cheaper analogue monitor, the infant then slept as well as they did with no monitor.

A DECT monitor placed in your baby's bedroom will expose them to more pulsing microwave radiation than living near to a mobile phone base station mast would do."

Alasdair Philips (2006) **(119)**

Radiation from baby monitors 'poses risk'

Infants being harmed by safety devices, say scientists

Baby monitors, bought by parents to keep their children safe, may instead be harming them, some scientists fear. They warn that the devices are bathing the infants in radiation at an age when they are most vulnerable to it.

Professor Denis Henshaw of the University of Bristol said the monitors are "being marketed without any checks and balances or even studies into their effects".

Dr Roger Coghill, who runs a laboratory specialising in the radiation, suggested that the DECT monitors should be placed at least 10 feet from infants. He said, "You want to hear what a baby is up to, but you don't want to harm him or her."

The Independent, *May 20, 2007* **(120)**

7.   *Unborn children need to be protected too*

Recent research has shown that pregnant mothers' phone use of mobile phones may have a direct effect on their children's emotional and behavioural development. It appears that even as few as two or three calls a day can make a difference.

The research showed that when the mothers of unborn babies were exposed to mobile phone radiation, their children had a far greater likelihood of being hyperactive and of displaying emotional and behavioural problems by the time they reached school age.

(See quote 102, from 'The Independent' *on page 148)*

> *"Pregnant women may also be at increased risk, based on a study showing that children born to mothers who used a cell phone just two or three times a day during pregnancy showed a dramatic increase in hyperactivity and other behavioral and emotional problems.*
>
> *And for the 30% of children who had also used a cell phone by age 7, the incidence of behavioral problems was 80% higher!"*
>
> **Paul J Rosch**   *(121)*

Even though this research concentrated on mobile phones, don't forget that cordless phones have the same effect.

Mothers-to-be can minimise their exposure and help to protect their children by making their calls on landlines with a corded handset.

> *"Pregnant women and children of all ages should avoid using cell and cordless phones given the health effects we are seeing already."*
>
> **Yuri Grigoriev** *(2011)* *(122)*

> *"Changes in the genes 'switched on' during a baby's development in the womb have also been described in rats that were exposed to a mobile phone during pregnancy.*
>
> *Which genes are 'switched on' determines how the baby develops.*
>
> *A research group in Saudi Arabia found that a mobile phone held close to the abdomen of pregnant women for ten minutes increased the baby's heart rate and decreased the amount of blood being pumped by the heart."*
>
> **Sarah J Starkey** *(2010)* *(123)*

Wi-Fi in Schools:
HOW IT CAN *PREVENT* LEARNING

The facts behind the concern about Wi-Fi in schools

> As we now know, installing a wireless system into a school or university fills the space with microwave radiation. This means that everyone working in that space - young children, teenagers, and teachers - is exposed to microwave radiation.

> This will be constant exposure - *all* the time, *every* time they are there.

> The concern is that this will considerably add to their cumulative exposure levels, making them feel unwell in the short term and potentially leading to ill health in the long term due to chronic exposure.

> For some children, this exposure may also lead to difficulties with learning, as well as changes in behaviour, moods, and social interaction.

"There is a great misconception that Wi-Fi in the public school system helps learning.

Wi-Fi disrupts learning. Wi-Fi causes ADD and ADHD in children.

Wi-Fi in schools means that these children and teachers are sitting for eight hours a day in a field of electromagnetic radiation with fields strong enough to carry the Internet."

Elizabeth Barris *(2009)* *(124)*

The potential health effects on school children

Due to the high number of hours children spend at school, constant exposure to wireless will substantially add to their overall accumulation of the effects of radiation exposure.

How this affects the child or teacher depends entirely on their own individual makeup, as does the time lag before they may experience any symptoms (physical, emotional, or behavioural).

> *"Our brains and nervous systems work by using electrical signals.*
>
> *I believe these signals are being interfered with by exposure to this Wi-Fi radiation."*
>
> *"Based on studies reporting effects experienced by people living near mobile phone masts, I would predict chronic fatigue, memory and concentration problems, irritability and behaviour problems - exactly what we are seeing increasingly in our school pupils. "*
>
> **Alasdair Philips** *(2007)* **(125)**

The more sensitive students and teachers are, the more likely they will *instantly* feel the effects of being exposed to wireless.

They may have:

- headaches,
- 'brain fog' - an inability to concentrate or think properly,
- nausea and dizziness,
- aggressive behaviour and mood swings,
- 'jitteriness' or an inability to keep calm and still,
- tiredness, and
- a general feeling of being 'spacey' or unwell'.

They may find that they feel better when they get home, only to have the symptoms reappear when they return to school.

166

Conversely, if there's wireless and/or a DECT cordless phone system installed in their home, then they may not find any relief there either.

"The Council of Europe is recommending that restrictions be put in place on the use of mobile phones and access to the Internet in all schools across the continent to protect young children from harmful radiation.

The recommendation is contained in a report on the potential dangers of electromagnetic fields and their effect on the environment drafted by Luxembourg Socialist MP Jean Huss, and adopted as a resolution by the Council of Europe's parliamentary assembly on 27 May."

British Medical Journal, *July 2011* **(126)**

"The ill health effects from the current wireless infrastructure effects both the students and teachers who are forced to work in a highly charged EMR environment.

A hard wired cable or DSL environment would give the same benefits of fast Internet access but without the ill health effects."

Elizabeth Barris *(2005)* **(127)**

> "It is unethical to expose children to electromagnetic load in this way.
>
> We know that power stations for electromagnetic waves like mobile phones are hurting the brains of children, so to put such stations into schools is really . . . very, very, very bad."
>
> "Does the school, or does the society, really want to have intelligent, well-educated children, or not?
>
> If you install mobile phone towers, which radiate to the children, their intelligence, their brain capacity, decreases.
>
> You will have more ADD children, you will have less function of the brain, which in the long term reflects on the intelligence of the children, of the possibility to really teach children, and in the long term, the more this overcomes society, the more we will have dumb children."
>
> **Thomas Rau** (2009) **(128)**

What can you do if your child goes to a school with Wi-Fi?

Talk to the parents' organisation at your school, and the school principal.

Educate them about the very real health concerns to children in schools with Wi-Fi.

Provide them with the evidence they'll need to make a decision - information and links - so that they can establish that your concerns are based on research and fact, and that your opinion is informed and educated

> *"I would recommend to parents to tell the school to remove Wi-Fi, and otherwise I would change the school even."*
>
> **Gerd Oberfeld** *(2007)* *(129)*

True duty of care means that both children and staff should be entitled to a safe working and learning environment. At the very least they should be able to safeguard their health by opting out of the blanket Wi-Fi policies implemented by schools.

Enough is now known about the potential health consequences to state that it is more than reasonable that they should be provided with access to Wi-Fi free-classrooms with cabled computers.

> *"Also do not forget the new EU recommendations about the 'producer's legal responsibility,' ie, in this case - since the school is producing the teaching - one must hold the school fully responsible for any negative, short- or long-term, effects.*
>
> *Lack of knowledge cannot be used as an excuse to use a certain technology."*
>
> **Olle Johansson** *(2005)* *(130)*

More information and help on Wi-Fi in Schools

Following are some websites with further information:

www.wifiinschools.org.uk/
www.wifiinschools.org.uk/resources/safeschools2012.pdf
www.wifiinschools.org.uk/resources/wireless+technologies+and+young+
people+Oct2011.pdf
www.safeschool.ca
www.citizensforsafetechnology.org
www.centerforsafewrwireless.org
www.emeffectsonkids.com
www.electricalpollution.com/documents/WiFischools09.pdf
www.wiredchild.org/schools.html
www.voicetheunion.org.uk/files/.../Wi-fiAdvicetoSchools0607.doc
www.emfacts.com/wifi/wlans_article.html
www.radiationeducation.com/home.html *(EMR Safety for kids, by kids)*

(There are also three valuable reports listed on page 208.)

"Based on the existing science, many public health experts believe it is possible we will face an epidemic of cancers in the future resulting from uncontrolled use of cell phones, and increased population exposure to Wi-Fi and other wireless devices.

Thus, it is important that all of us, and especially children, restrict our use of cell phones, limit exposure to background levels of Wi-Fi, and that government and industry discover ways in which to allow use of wireless devices without such elevated risk of serious disease. We need to educate decision-makers that 'business as usual' is unacceptable."

David O Carpenter *(131)*

Dr Andrew Goldsworthy on Wi-Fi in Schools

It was first shown by Bawin et al. in the 1970s that weak amplitude modulated radio waves, where the strength of the signal rises and falls at low frequencies, could remove some of this calcium from brain cell membranes. This destabilises them and make them more likely to leak. The low frequency pulsations of Wi-Fi and mobile phone signals can be expected to behave in much the same way.

This is important in the brain because the normal function of brain cells depends on the controlled passage of specific ions through their membranes. When these membranes leak, ions flow through them in a relatively uncontrolled way, which results in brain hyperactivity and may cause attention deficit hyperactivity disorder (ADHD) in some people.

When this occurs in the brain of a foetus or very young child it prevents normal brain development, which may result in autism. (See http:// mcs-america.org/june2011pg2345.pdf).

Wi-Fi should therefore be considered as an impediment rather than an aid to learning and may be particularly hazardous for pregnant teachers.

Effects on the peripheral nervous system are equally damaging since hyperactivity here causes false sensations such as pain, heat, cold, and pins and needles in some people (i.e., symptoms of electromagnetic hypersensitivity). Hyperactivity in the cells of the inner ear can cause tinnitus and affect the sense of balance causing dizziness and symptoms of motion sickness, including nausea.

Pupils showing any of these symptoms should be treated with sympathy and the Wi-Fi switched off . . .

Fortunately, because of genetic variability, not everyone will suffer the same symptoms and many may suffer none at all; but for the sake of those that do suffer, Wi-Fi is not a good idea in schools, or anywhere else for that matter.

Andrew Goldsworthy (2011) **(132)**

"Revealed - radiation threat from new wireless computer networks"

Teachers demand inquiry to protect a generation of pupils.

"Britain's top health protection watchdog is pressing for a formal investigation into the hazards of using wireless communication networks in schools amid mounting concern that they may be damaging children's health.

Sir William Stewart, the chairman of the Health Protection Agency, wants pupils to be monitored for ill effects from the networks - known as Wi-Fi - which emit radiation and are being installed in classrooms across the nation.

Professor Olle Johansson, of Sweden's prestigious Karolinska Institute, who is deeply concerned about the spread of Wi-Fi, says there are "thousands" of articles in scientific literature demonstrating "adverse health effects".

He adds: "Do we not know enough already to say, 'Stop!?'"

The Independent; April 22, 2007 *(133)*

Supplements That Protect Against EMR-Induced Damage

Something that really stands out when you read the research on EMR exposure is the extent to which oxidative stress is mentioned. Oxidative stress is linked to cellular damage, degeneration, and ageing.

Doing all you can to counter this oxidative stress helps you to protect yourself against EMR exposure, and take back some control of your health. One of the most effective tools is the use of antioxidants, of which there are many sources.

Specific studies on the following have found them to be protective against the effects of EMR exposure.

Vitamin C	**Ginko Biloba**	**Garlic**
Vitamin E	**Selenium**	**L-carnitine**
Melatonin	**Green Tea**	

It goes without saying that, if you can, getting these through your diet is preferable. A diet high in a wide variety of fresh fruit and vegetables (preferably organic) is highly beneficial. They will not only make you feel great, but are all naturally packed full of antioxidants, and a variety of other components that are protective of health.

Sometimes it's not possible to get everything we need through our diet, so supplements can be very useful. However, be mindful that we all have individual reactions to supplements. Sometimes our bodies can be intolerant of them, or doses can be too high for us. It's also possible that they may interact with each other, or with any medication that's being taken.

As always, research well (particularly side effects). And above all, *listen to your own body.*

(Research into these supplements is listed on pages 295-7 in the 'Research Studies' section of 'Hold the Phone: Here's Why'.)

Top Tips To Remember
about phones and wireless

The most urgent priorities
for minimising exposure are:

1. Avoid putting the phone next to your head.

2. Avoid 'wearing' it on your body.

3. Replace cordless phones with corded ones.

4. Use cabled/corded computers (and other devices).

5. Keep all devices away from you when you're sleeping.

6. Make sure that children are kept away from phones and wireless.

7. . . . and also pregnant women and their unborn children.

"Unthinking respect for authority
is the greatest enemy of truth."

Albert Einstein

PART 2

WHAT THE RESEARCH HAS FOUND

Phones and 'Wireless'

The research

"At most, recognizing that our history was inspired by many tales we now recognize as false should make us alert, ready to call to constantly into question the very tale we believe true. . .

. . .because the criterion of the wisdom of the community is based on constant awareness of the fallibility of our learning."

Umberto Eco

Research Headlines

What the Research Actually Says

Given on the following pages are just a few examples of the findings from some of the research studies on the radiation that's emitted by mobile phones, cordless phones and all devices 'wireless'.

The full story about the amount of this research – and the effects of the radiation - is covered in the companion book *'Hold the Phone: Here's Why'*.

Also shared in this follow-up book are details of some of the more important research.

These are studies that have found links between varying forms of wireless technology and biological changes, and also adverse effects on health.

These effects were observed to range from the physical, mental, and emotional to behavioural.

The studies are presented for you - listed by symptom - so that you can easily see, just by thumbing through the pages, just *how much* research has found an effect - and also the various forms in which these effects present in people.

Research into this highly complex subject is constantly changing and evolving. Following are highlights of some of the research to date . . .

Brain Tumours

Cell phone use increases the likelihood of brain tumours

1   *Cell phone use causes brain tumours: (1)*
- *A statistically significant doubling of brain cancer risk*
- *A statistically significant dose-response risk of acoustic*
- *neuroma with more than six years of cell phone use, plus*
- *Findings of genetic damage in human blood when exposed to cell phone radiation*

2   *"The results indicate that using a cell phone for more than ten years approximately doubles the risk of being diagnosed with a brain tumor on the same side of the head as that preferred for cell phone use." (2)*

3   *A "significantly increased" risk of brain tumors from 10 or more years of cell phone or cordless phone use. Among their many significant findings are the following: (3)*
- *For every 100 hours of cell phone use, the risk of brain cancer increases by 5%.*
- *For every year of cell phone use, the risk of brain cancer increases by 8%.*
- *After 10 or more years of digital cell phone use, there was a 280% increased risk of brain cancer.*
- *For digital cell phone users who were teenagers or younger when they first started using a cell phone, there was a 420% increased risk of brain cancer."*
- *Cordless phone users, when use began as teenagers or younger, there was a 340% increased risk.*

"Because the latency between exposure and brain cancer could be 20 or 30 years . . .

. . . we are basically treating ourselves like lab rats in an experiment without any controls."

Devra Lee Davis *(2009)* **(134)**

> *"All the independently-funded studies that included longer term users (10 years or more use) have shown an association between brain tumour incidence and mobile phone use. In a number of studies the risks for some types of tumours is doubled or even quadrupled.*
>
> *(The only studies that have not shown such a link were funded by the mobile phone industry, or only analysed short-term duration of use.")*
>
> **Wired Child** *(135)*

Reduced Health

Health Effects of Cell Phone Use

1. *Prolonged mobile phone use (more than 25 min/day for two weeks) was associated with a reduction in the concentration of the hormone melatonin in adults. (4)*

2. *Cell phone use affects the brain: Exposure to GSM signal for forty-five minutes modified inter-hemispheric EEG coherence in the brain. (5)*

3. *Studies have reported that as short as a single, two-hour exposure to cell phone radiation will result in pathological leakage of the blood brain barrier. The effect occurs immediately and is still seen at fourteen days and at fifty days post-exposure. (6)*

4. *"These results highlight a correlation between mobile phone use and genetic damage." (7)*

5. *"It appears that MRI and microwave radiation emitted from mobile phones significantly releases mercury from dental amalgam restoration." (8)*

6. *"Results showed that the RFR exposure significantly increased DNA double-strand breaks in brain cells." (9)*

7. *Exposure to pulsed modulated RFR prior to sleep altered cerebral blood flow and affected EEG during sleep. (10)*

8. *RF exposure resulted in prolonged time to reach deep (stage 3) and shortened deep (stages 3 and 4) sleep. "If you have trouble sleeping, you should think about not talking on a mobile phone right before you go to bed." (11)*

9. *"Mobile phone radiation might cause Alzheimer's disease after approximately 10 years of use. The mortality in Alzheimer's disease appears to be associated with mobile phone output power. The mortality is increasing fast and is expected to increase substantially within the next 10 years." (12)*

Headaches and Migraines

Increase in Migraines and Vertigo

1 *A study of 420,000 adults in Denmark showed that long-term mobile phone users were 10-20% more likely to be hospitalized for migraines and vertigo than people who'd more recently started using a phone. (13)*

Pregnancy

The effect on women using cell phones during pregnancy

1 *A giant study, surveying more than 13,000 children, found that their mothers' use of cell phones during pregnancy led to their babies developing hyperactivity by the time they reached school age, along with difficulties with conduct, emotions, and relationships.*

2. *Using the phones only two or three times a day was enough to increase the risk (by 80%). The likelihood increased if the children themselves used the phones before the age of seven. (14)*

3. *A ten- minute exposure to a mobile phone during pregnancy significantly increased the heart rate of the unborn baby, and significantly decreased the amount of blood being pumped by its heart. Exposure after birth had the same effect on the newborn. (15)*

Children

Children are particularly vulnerable to the radiation from cell phones

1.   Scientists have discovered that a call lasting just two minutes can alter the natural electrical activity of a child's brain for up to an hour afterwards. (16)

2.   In children reporting more mobile phone voice calls, the accuracy of working memory was poorer. (17)

3.   Several studies report that the brains of children absorb more radiation than those of adults. (18)

Fertility

Cell phone use and reduced fertility in males

1.   Exposure of human sperm in vitro to a mobile phone for five minutes significantly decreased sperm motility. (19)

2.   RFR from mobile phones decreases the motility and vitality of human sperm cells while stimulating DNA fragmentation. "These findings have clear implications for the safety of extensive mobile phone use by males of reproductive age, potentially affecting both their fertility and the health and wellbeing of their offspring." (20)

Phone Masts and Antenna

Living close to Phone Masts: The Link with Cancer

1.   Cancers were significantly higher (three times) among those who had lived for ten years within four hundred metres of the cell phone mast, compared with those living further away. The patients had fallen ill on average eight years earlier. (21)

2.   "This first study on symptoms experienced by people living in vicinity of base stations shows that the minimal distance of people from cellular phone base stations should not be less than three hundred meters." (22)

Addiction
The possible mechanism behind cell phone addiction?

1.   *"Low-level RF activates both endogenous opioids and other substances in the brain that function in a similar manner to psychoactive drug actions. Such effects in laboratory animals mimic the effects of drugs on the part of the brain that is involved in addiction." (23)*

(All these studies are listed in 'Research Headlines - References' on page 234.)

And so, just *how much* research has there been?

There have been many thousands of research studies conducted.

And – contrary to what you may well have heard - thousands of these studies *have* found evidence of biological changes and health effects.

Take a look over the next three pages, as they will give you the merest glimpse into only a few of the studies that have taken place – and the wide range of symptoms that have been shown to occur after exposure to radio frequency/microwave radiation.

Please remember: this is nowhere near a complete list.   This only represents a portion of the studies that have found effects.

"Fear grows in the darkness.
If you think there's a bogeyman around, turn on the light."
                                                        Dorothy Thompson

THE RESEARCH STUDIES:

AN INDEX

How mobile phones, cordless phones, wireless technology, and microwave radiation can affect biology and health

Here's a brief list of just *some* of the studies that are listed in more detail in *'Hold the Phone: Here's Why'*.

They are listed here by the health effect that was linked to the exposure to mobile phones and/or radio frequency radiation.

They represent only a small sample of the research.

Symptom/Effect	No of Studies
Acoustic neuroma (type of benign brain tumour)	21
Addiction to mobile phones	18
Agitation, hyperactivity, tremors	7
Anxiety, nervousness	16
Autism	3
Behaviour (changes to)	35
Biology and biological processes	205
Blood flow and composition (changes to)	50
Blood brain barrier (permeability)	27
Blood pressure, high (hypertension)	8
Blood sugar, insulin, diabetes	5

Symptom/Effect	No of Studies
Bones and bone marrow	12
Brain (changes to processes/function)	189
Brain cancer, brain tumours	58
Cancer and carcinogenesis	49
Cancer - Breast cancer	9
Cancer - Childhood	12
Cancer - Leukaemia	18
Cancer - Lymphoma	8
Cancer - Melanoma, Skin cancer	14
Cancer - Testicular cancer	6
Children (increased risk, and damage to)	61
CNS (central nervous system affected)	28
Depression	14
Dizziness, light-headedness, and vertigo	17
Driving (increased accident rate)	11
Ears, hearing, and tinnitus	27
Electrosensitivity (sensitivity to EMR)	26
Epilepsy and seizures	9
Eyes and vision	57
Fatigue, tiredness, and exhaustion	24
Genetic damage (DNA breaks, inhibited DNA repair)	91
Headaches and migraine	36
Heart (and cardiovascular system)	24
Heart (effect on pacemakers)	7
Hormones and endocrine system	24
Immune system, immune function	35
Irritability and aggression	11
Kidneys	6
Learning (attention, concentration, cognition)	55

Symptom/Effect	No of Studies
Liver	8
Melatonin production, impaired	15
Memory	39
Mortality and decreased lifespan	15
Nature - Animals and insects	13
Nature - Plants	14
Oxidative stress and damage	55
Pain, aches, and discomfort	27
Reaction time (slower response)	16
Reproduction (changes to, difficulty with)	21
Reproduction (issues with female fertility)	6
Reproduction (issues with male fertility)	60
Reproduction - Prenatal (effects on pregnancy/fetus)	49
Skin	15
Sleep	48
Weakness	4
Weight (significant weight gain)	2
Wellbeing (reduced: feeling sick, general 'ill health')	22
Occupational Exposure	*45*
Supplements - protective effects	*32*

This is only a very small selection of the thousands of studies that have shown biological and other health effects of exposure to this type of radiation. Even if you have just the quickest flick through, do take look at the studies listed in the companion book: *'Hold the Phone: Here's Why'*.

You'll very quickly begin to understand the huge range of evidence that's been accumulated, and why the experts are trying so hard to warn you to take precautions.

Part 3

Where to now ?

THE WAY FORWARD

WHERE TO NOW?

*"The great thing in the world is not so much where we stand,
as in what direction we are moving."*

Oliver Wendell Holmes

To sum up: What we fear vs what we know

There are many different scenarios being laid out for us at the moment. From head-in-the-sand denials to alarmist reportage, the 'advice' that you'll be subject to is very polarising. And much of it induces fear.

The truth of the matter - at the moment - is that no one can tell you exactly what the final outcome of this, the world's biggest ever in-field experiment, will be.

We will learn more with time; but right now, we just don't know how far-reaching the effects will be.

If you decide to research further, you'll come across many who hold the opinion that we may be heading for an epidemic of ill health as the result of our exposure to this radiation. Others believe that some of us can withstand it. We may even adapt. We don't know.

A percentage of people, usually those who are more sensitive, are already displaying symptoms. But not everyone is. The epidemic that's feared may be taking longer to happen than was first thought. Or it may not be going to happen at all. Again, we just don't know.

However, the research and trends do show us there are very real concerns about:

➢ the impact of the many forms of mobile telecommunications technology,

➢ the unrestrained way in which its widespread rollout has been unleashed onto an unsuspecting public around the world, the health effects it is already having on people,

➢ the potential scale and ramifications of health effects into the future

➢ especially on our children,

There is an urgent need for appropriate health-based safety standards, and for further independently funded research.

Everything you read about here is preventable

Ultimately, we must remember that mobile communications technology - and its resultant radiation - is here because of enhanced convenience.

The mobile companies marketed that convenience to us and we, in our billions, have gone along with their offer. Not only that we, the consumers, have given the telcos a mandate to continually expand their networks by demanding from them ever-increasing coverage and enhanced reception.

We really didn't understand the ramifications of that. (Most still don't.) But now we need to.

We must never lose sight of the fact that all this is preventable. We still have the power and the ability to choose health over convenience.

As individuals, we have choices within our own homes. We can easily choose to opt for wires and cables over the health risks of wireless. As communities, we can choose to work together to make our local environments safer for ourselves, our children, our grandchildren, and beyond.

As citizens of a country, we can collaborate and unite to put pressure on governments and corporations to prioritise health over profits – and to provide us with safer technology.

And even though the infrastructure and hardware that keeps us all enveloped within a blanket of radiation is in place, it is still not too late.

Whilst antennae and masts criss-cross our cities, counties, and countryside (and even our skies), they radiate only because they are programmed to do so. Just because the antennae are there does not mean that they have to continue to radiate. They can be turned off.

In reality, it is possible to reverse our levels of exposure. We just need to make the collective choice to make that happen.

WHAT IS THE PRECAUTIONARY PRINCIPLE?

The precautionary principle states:

> *"When there is reasonable suspicion of harm*
> *lack of scientific certainty or consensus*
> *must not be used to postpone preventative action."*

There is much, **much** more than enough evidence to show us that this radiation can and does affect health.

It's important to be both informed and careful; and to avoid exposure wherever and whenever it's possible to do so.

Many scientists, public health advocates, and doctors around the world are calling for the invocation of the precautionary principle in relation to EMR.

The first step in this is to advise everyone of the implications of using phones and wireless. That's the impetus behind this book: information on what to do so that we can all take remedial action. Now.

The second step is to stop the roll-out of yet further blanket coverage of cell phone, wireless, and Wi-Max antennae - especially if they are anywhere near our children.

What we DO know now:

There's enough evidence
to say that it's wise to take precautions.

WHAT TO DO?

What you can do personally:

Take action:

This book shows you *what* you can do to help yourself.

Educate yourself:

The companion book, *Hold The Phone: Here's Why*, explains why you need to be careful. By understanding this now, you can play it safe and take steps to protect your future, and that of your family.

Educate others:

Then pass the word on to your friends. This is something we all need to be talking about. And who better to start the conversation in your part of the world than you? Whether at the water cooler, the school gates, over dinner or on your blog, start your own ripple in the pond.

Become an agent for change:

Get involved with the many groups around the world who are doing what they can to convince governments and corporations of the need for reduced exposure levels – together with more research and biologically-based safety guidelines.

What we can do collectively:

Most importantly:

➢ We need to 'hold the phone' on the rapid and indiscriminate way in which this technology is being foisted on an uninformed public.

➢ We especially need to protect the most vulnerable members of our society: babies, yet-to-be-born babies, young children, and teenagers.

To do this, we simultaneously need to:

➢ Question the degree to which we adopt this technology (even while acknowledging that it does offer great advantages).

➢ Call a moratorium on the increasing global rollout of devices that bathe all those in their path in high frequency radiation. WiMAX and Wi-Fi in schools are prime examples. In both cases, individual needs have been ignored and personal choice has been removed.

➢ Pressure our governments for safer technology (such as fibre optics)

➢ Challenge our governing bodies (local and national) and schools further on the question of their duty of care (legally and morally).

➢ Start educating our doctors about the possible health effects of this radiation so that they can recognize the symptoms in their patients and advise them on what to do.

➢ Make public the possible health effects so that everyone has the ability to make an informed decision as to the degree to which they wish to participate in this experiment.

➢ Supply more alternatives for those who don't.

"Liberty cannot be preserved without general knowledge among people."

John Adams

Action and enquiry instead of fear

One of the reasons this book hasn't concentrated on the doom-laden forecasts is that engendering fear is always, always counterproductive.

Fear shuts us down. It triggers our sympathetic nervous system and kicks us right into 'fight or flight' response. This turns us into rabbits in the headlights and forces our systems into 'sympathetic lock.' And when we're in that state, we're in no condition to take in any meaningful information whatsoever. We can't hear, understand, recall, or process anything properly.

To take in information and learn, your mind needs to be open. No matter how hard you try, your mind is incapable of remaining open if it's being filled with fear.

So whatever you hear or read, do all you can to avoid going into a fear response. It won't help you. Nor will ignoring the issue. Remaining calm, becoming more informed, and taking action *will*.

The most helpful thing for you to focus on is not the future - not what *could* happen - but the present. Right now, find out what you can do to help yourself. And then just do it. Every little step you take will help to reduce your cumulative exposure levels and protect your health.

> "*I would like to see a change . . . a recognition that when you have a new industry with a product where the risk is uncertain, where science can't tell you that it's safe, and there is evidence that it may be harmful, that you err on the side of precaution. That you implement the patents, that you tell people what the risk is.*"
>
> *Carl Hilliard* (2005) *(136)*

HOW TO AVOID THE TWIN TRAPS
OF DENIAL AND DISSONANCE

When we acquire information that conflicts with our current world view, one of two things may happen to us: cognitive dissonance or denial.

Understanding these two will help you to assimilate what you've just read, and to better grasp what's happening when others are dismissive, resistant, or don't seem to 'get it'.

Cognitive dissonance is the mental conflict that occurs when our beliefs or assumptions are contradicted by new information.

This is particularly the case when we find out that the way we've led our life up to that moment has been based on falsehoods or incorrect assumptions. Our brain finds it difficult to reconcile the gap between what we thought was real and reality as we now understand it to be.

Having our eyes opened to the way things really are is not always a comfortable process.

When we realize that something we previously held to be a fundamental truth no longer holds water, it can leave us on shaky ground. The moment we accept the newer version of reality, our lives will have to change. And often that very thought fills us with fear.

Humans generally like the status quo. We seem to dislike change, especially if it is substantial and uninvited (not of our choosing). When something comes along that threatens to change our way of life, we tend to do all we can to prevent that change. (This can happen on conscious or subconscious levels.)

We may try to:

➢ explain away the information,

➢ Google frantically to find an alternative viewpoint (one that will concur with our current way of being)

- ➤ convince ourselves this simply can't be so - much easier to do when there are billions behaving just like us (the 'million flies can't be wrong' argument),

- ➤ avoid the information (the 'ostrich' approach), or

- ➤ reject the information outright.

One common way of preventing new information from changing your life is by dismissing it. By going into denial, one can simply close down, block out the news, and attempt to keep on keeping on.

I have seen people, friends even, who upon hearing this information have taken a moment to think, shaken their heads, and then simply said "No!". End of discussion.

When we deny things, we're blocking an external influence from entering into our awareness. If the news is just too much for us to handle, we attempt to avoid entering into the experience by refusing to accept that it's happening. But that doesn't change reality. It is still there. No matter how hard we try, we're not able to change the event, or the truth. However, what we *can* change is our ability to accept what is. And then find a solution, and act upon it.

New, challenging information can either hit you like a lightning bolt (an epiphany where you instantly realise that it's 'right'), or the news can take a while to sink in. Sometimes you just need the space to go over the facts time and time again, until eventually the mist clears and you see things in a different light.

Because this information comes in the form of a set of books, you have the opportunity to go over it repeatedly - page by page, in your own time, as much and as often as you need to assimilate what's there. Give yourself time to let the dust settle, time for it all to sink in. And then make up your own mind about where reality really lies.

"One reason we resist making deliberate choices is that choice equals change and most of us, feeling the world is unpredictable enough, try to minimise the trauma of change in our personal lives."

Hugh Mackay

LET'S BE CLEAR: *SAFER* STILL DOESN'T MEAN 'SAFE'

We've come to think of our cell phones as mere communication devices. As you now know, the truth is far more stark; they emit microwave radiation which research is showing us can fundamentally alter our biology, and has the very real potential to damage our health.

Because of this, no one can tell you that it's safe to use a mobile phone.

We need to be very clear here. The very best strategy in protecting your health from mobile phone radiation is simply not to use them. The same applies to cordless phones and all things 'wireless.'

In terms of health, the best connection is a wired one.

The cables, cords and wires used within wired technology encase the radiation and help to isolate it, leading it from point to point with the smallest chance of human exposure. They may not offer you the ultimate in aesthetics - or convenience - but they do offer you your best chance of good health. They are the safest choice.

Being pragmatic, the important thing here is to offer practical help to those who do choose to continue to use this technology – and realistically that's likely to be the overwhelming majority.

Because there is a potential risk to your health associated with wireless phones and devices, if you choose to keep using them, then your priority needs to become *risk minimisation.*

The experts' advice is to **reduce your exposure as much as you possibly can**. The usage tips in this book will show the very best ways of doing that, so you can minimise the risks to your health.

However, it's very important to understand that while following these tips will make it 'safer' to use your mobile phone, they still can't make it 'safe'.

So, to sum up:
How do you protect your health while staying connected?

To stay safe, you need to use cables, cords, and wires.
That is the very best advice there is.

What presents to you now is a simple choice: Your health? Or convenience?

Knowledge is power. And having read this, you are now informed enough to make that decision.

The decision is very individual. Not everyone's will take the choice that's best for their health.

The important thing to remember is: Now you do *have* a choice.

"Every choice you make has an end result."

Zig Ziglar

Part 4

Where to find more information

IF YOU'D LIKE TO
KNOW MORE . . .

The following all offer a comprehensive insight into the issues surrounding mobile telecommunications and the effects of electro-pollution.

Reading any of them will significantly help you to gain further understanding into the issues surrounding the use of cell phones, cordless phones, wireless, and wireless in schools.

"Gather experience . . .
Look at what you should not look at.
A feeling of anxiety is the sure and certain evidence that you should do this."

Clive Barker

BOOKS: (In no particular order)

Cell Phones: Invisible Hazards in the Wireless Age: An Insider's Alarming Discoveries about Cancer and Genetic Damage. George Carlo and Martin Schram. Basic Books, 2002.

Cell Towers: Wireless Convenience? or Environmental Hazard? B Blake Levitt. Safe Goods, 2001.

The Powerwatch Handbook: Simple Ways to Make Your Environment Safer. Alasdair and Jean Philips. Piatkus Books, 2006.

The Invisible Disease: The Dangers of Environmental Illnesses Caused by Electromagnetic Fields and Chemical Emissions. Gunni Nordström. O Books, 2004.

Electropollution: How to Protect Yourself Against It. Roger Coghill. Thorsons Publishing, 1990.

Cross Currents: The Perils of Electropollution, the Promise of Electromedicine. Robert O Becker. Tarcher, 1990.

iDisorder: Understanding Our Obsession with Technology and Overcoming Its Hold on Us. Larry D Rosen. Palgrae Macmillan, 2012.

Warning: The electricity around you may be hazardous to your health. Ellen Sugarman. MiriamPress, 2004.

Public Health SOS: The Shadow Side of the Wireless Revolution. Camilla Rees and Magda Havas. Create Space Independent Publishing Platform, 2009.

Would You Put Your Head in a Microwave Oven? Gerald Goldberg. AuthorHouse, 2006.

Zapped: Why Your Cell Phone Shouldn't Be Your Alarm Clock, and 1268 Ways to Outsmart the Hazards of Electronic Pollution. Ann Louise Gittleman. HarperOne, 2011.

The Force: Living Safely in a World of Electromagnetic Pollution. Lyn McLean. Scribe Publications, 2011.

Disconnect: The Truth About Cell Phone Radiation, What the Industry is Doing to Hide It, and How to Protect Your Family.   Devra Davis. Plume, 2011.

Cellular Telephone Russian Roulette. Robert C Kane. Vantage Pr, 2001.

Cell Phones and the Dark Deception: Find Out What You're Not Being Told . . . And Why. Carleigh Cooper. Premier Advantage Publishing, 2009.

The Electrical Sensitivity Handbook: How Electromagnetic Fields (EMFs) Are Making People Sick. Lucinda Grant. Weldon Publishing, 1995.

ARTICLES, LETTERS, AND REPORTS

Carlo, George:

Illusion and Escape: The Cell Phone Disease Quagmire.
A Summary of American Legal Actions Regarding Mobile Phones and Health Effects
www.naturalscience.org/fileadmin/portabledocuments/fact_sheet_no_01.pdf

Letter to Maine Legislature. SPPI. March 2010.
www.scribd.com/doc/28894870/Letter-to-Maine-Legislature-Regarding-Warning-Label-Bill

Goldsworthy, Andrew:

Comments by Andrew Goldsworthy on Health Protection Agency Press Release entitled "Scientist probe laptops Wi-Fi Emissions". September 2009
www.radiationresearch.org/pdfs/20090926_hpa_wifi_ag_comments.pdf

Wi-Fi in Schools
www.emfacts.com/2011/11/dr-andrew-goldsworthy-on-wi-fi-in-schools/

Andrew Goldsworthy Witness Statement, April 2010
www.mastsanity.org/health/research/292-dr-andrew-goldsworthy-witness-statement-april-2010.html

Hemingway, Patty:

The risks to health from pulsed microwaves
An interview with Ingrid Dickenson, Homeopathy in practice, Spring 2006.
*www.buergerwelle.de/assets/files/the_risk_to_health_from_pulsed_microwaves.
pdf?cultureKey=&q=pdf/the_risk_to_health_from_pulsed_microwaves.pdf*

What to do when electro-smog makes you sick
Homeopathy in practice, Summer 2006
www.a-r-h.org/Publications/Journal/BackIssues.htm

Ketcham, Christopher:

Warning: Your Cell Phone May Be Hazardous to Your Health
GQ Magazine, Feburary 2010
www.gq.com/cars-gear/gear-and-gadgets/201002/warning-cell-phone-radiation

Khurana, Vini:

Mobile Phones and Brain Tumours - A Public Health Concern
www.brain-surgery.us/mobph.pdf

Maisch, Don:

*Children and mobile phones: Is there a health risk? The case for extra
precautions*
J Aust Coll Nutr & Env Med Vol 22 No 2 August 2003
www.emfacts.com/papers/

Medical warnings needed on DECT cordless phone use
J Aust Coll Nutr & Env Med Vol 25 No 2 August 2006
www.emfacts.com/papers/

Mobile Phone Use: It's time to take precautions
J Aust Coll Nutr & Env Med Vol 20 No 1 April 2001
www.emfacts.com/papers/

Morgan, L Lloyd: (Primary Author and Main Editor)

*Cellphones and Brain Tumors: 15 Reasons for Concern:
Science, Spin and the Truth Behind Interphone*
www.radiationresearch.org/pdfs/reasons_a4.pdf

Phillips, Alasdair and Jean: (Powerwatch)

Children and Mobile Phones: Parts 1–3

1. *www.powerwatch.org.uk/library/downloads/children-phones-1-use-2012-03.pdf*
2. *www.powerwatch.org.uk/library/downloads/children-phones-2-advice-2012-09.pdf*
3. *www.powerwatch.org.uk/library/downloads/children-phones-3-research-2012-03.pdf*

Reports available to subscribers:

1. *"Radiofrequency Protection for You and Your Family"*
   www.powerwatch.org.uk

2. *"Electrical Hypersensitivity, A Modern Illness"*
   www.powerwatch.org.uk

3. *"Radiofrequency EMF's and Health"*
   www.powerwatch.org.uk

4. *"Mobile Phones"* *www.powerwatch.org.uk*

Starkey, Sarah:

Living in a Wireless World
For the National Childbirth Trust. January 2010.
www.cavisoc.org.uk/National%20Childbirth%20Trust%20Jan%202010.pdf

Other Reports:

The BioInitiative Reports (2007 and 2012)
A Rationale for publically based Public Exposure Standards for EM Fields (ELF and RF).
www.bioinitiative.org/report/index.htm

The Cell Phone Problem
Cell Phones: Technology, Exposures, Health Effects
www.ehhi.org/reports/cellphones/cell_phone_report_EHHI_Feb2012.pdf

ICEMS - International Commission on Electromagnetic Safety
Campaign for Safer Cell Phone Use
www.icems.eu/public_education.htm

Joining the Dots
An Overview of Public Health Trends in 2007. Australian Democrats
www.democrats.org.au/docs/2007/Joining_the_Dots11.pdf

Mobilewise
Mobile phone health risks: the case for action to protect children
www.mobilewise.org/wordpress/wp-content/uploads/MobileWise_mobile_phone_health_risks_NEW.pdf

Wi-Fi in Schools:

Safe Schools 2012: Medical and Scientific Experts Call For Safe Technologies in Schools. A document for schools.
www.wifiinschools.org.uk/resources/safeschools2012.pdf

Wireless Devices, Standards, and Microwave radiation in the Education Environment. Gary Brown, October 2000.
www.getpurepower.ca/resources/WireleassDevices_GaryBrown.pdf

Wireless technologies and young people: A resource for schools.
Wifiinschools.org.uk, October 2011
www.wifiinschools.org.uk/resources/wireless+technologies+and+young+people+Oct2011.pdf

YouTube

1. *BBC Panorama. Wi-Fi: A Warning Signal.*

   a. Part 1: *www.youtube.com/watch?v=IuNaDj6VLHw*
   b. Part 2: *www.youtube.com/watch?v=yQGo0hesqIg&feature=relmfu*
   c. Part 3: *www.youtube.com/watch?v=VqnPtq4GbU*

2. *Larry King Live: Cell Phone Dangers*
   www.youtube.com/watch?v=yKHg08f5_xo

3. *Wi-Fi in Schools.*
   www.youtube.com/watch?v=IgLO9yR1JlQ

4. *Wi-Fi in Schools is Proven Dangerous. www.youtube.com/
   watch?v=KN7VetsCR2I*

5. *Cell Phone War*
   Part 1: *www.youtube.com/watch?v=sEqCkwPmQ_w*

6. *Public Exposure: DNA, Democracy and the 'Wireless Revolution'*
   Part 1: *www.youtube.com/watch?v=IjbCa-MZwXM*

7. *Olle Johansson: Is it safe or not?* (In 15 parts)
   Part 1: *www.youtube.com/watch?v=eS7YIZ1x0r8*

8. *Dangers of cell phone wi-fi radiation - George Carlo.*

   a. Part 1: *www.youtube.com/watch?v=kofG4W74tIE*
   b. Part 2: *www.youtube.com/watch?v=Urzibz5_CyQ*
   c. Part 3: *www.youtube.com/watch?v=YHVaK0Ih08c*

Radio Interviews

'Your Own Health and Fitness'.
Radio Show with Jeffry Fawcett and Layna Berman

The following interviews (and others) are available for download from:
www.yourownhealthandfitness.org/?page_id=753

1. "Health Considerations for the Digital Revolution" with B Blake Levitt
2. "Industry Censored Cell Phone Science" with Devra Davis
3. "Wireless Risks in the Mainstream" with Christopher Ketcham and Michael Segell
4. "Wireless Technology Health News" with Cindy Sage
5. "Alternatives to Wireless broadband" with Doug Loranger and Sally Hampton
6. "Secondhand Cell Phone Radiation" with Cindy Sage
7. "Hypersensitivity," a discussion
8. "Wi-Max, the Next Wireless Exposure" with Libby Kelley
9. "The Science of RFR Health Risks" with Olle Johansson
10. "Wireless Public Health Crisis" with B Blake Levitt, Jan Newton, and Doug Loranger
11. "Cell Phones and Breast Cancer" with John West

Documentary DVDs:

Resonance: Beings of Frequency. A James Russell film; Flat Frog Productions, 2012. *www.flatfrogfilms.com/resonance-documentary/*

Full Signal: The Hidden Cost of Cellphones.
Directed by Talal Jabari. *www.fullsignalmovie.com*

Cell Phone War.
Filmmaker Klaus Scheidsteger. DVD of documentary aired on French TV, 2005.

Public Exposure: DNA, Democracy and the Wireless Revolution.
Co-produced by EON, The Ecological Options Network and the Council on Wireless Technology Impacts.

Websites

The following are websites with information that may be useful to you in your further research on the health effects of mobile phones, cordless phones, and wireless.

Recommended Web sites: (listed alphabetically)

www.bioinitiative.org

www.buergerwelle.de/body_science.html

www.buergerwelle.de/en/

www.electromagnetichealth.org

www.emfacts.com

www.icems.eu

www.microwavenews.com

www.powerwatch.org.uk

www.radiationeducation.com
www.safertech.com
www.weepinitiative.org

Electrosensitivity Web sites:

www.electrosensitivity.co.uk
www.electrosensitivity.org
www.electrosensitivesociety.com/
www.es-uk.info
www.org.feb.nu/index_int.htm
www.weepinitiative.org/livingwithEHS.html

Children and Wi-Fi in Schools Web sites:

www.citizensforsafetechnology.org
www.radiationeducation.com
www.safeinschool.org/
www.safeschool.ca/
www.ssita.org.uk
www.wifiinschools.org.uk
www.wiredchild.org

Other Web sites of interest:

www.bemri.org
www.brain-surgery.us/mobilephone.html
www.cavisoc.org.uk

www.cellphonetaskforce.org

www.centerforsaferwireless.org/Home.php

www.emfbioeffects.org

www.emrnetwork.org

www.emrpolicy.org

www.emrstop.org

www.ideaireland.org/emr.htm

www.mastaction.co.uk

www.mastsanity.org

www.mast-victims.org

www.neilcherry.com

www.notowersnearschools.com

www.psrast.org/mobileng/mobilstarteng.htm

www.radiationresearch.org

www.rewire.me

www.stop-radiation.com/

www.tetrawatch.net

Resources:

Training Courses and Professional Help

Courses on Electrosmog and Healthy Homes

The International Institute for Building-Biology and Ecology (IBE): This was my starting point when I wanted to learn all I could about how to create a healthy home.

General Interest Courses:

The IBE has many general interest courses for people who just want to learn more about how to make their own home healthy. These are short online courses, many of which are free. The subjects offered include Intro to Electrosmog, Healthy Nursery, Nursery Electrosmog, Sleeping Sanctuary, and Cell Phones. Further information about all their training courses is available at *www.hbelc.org/courses.html.* (They often hold conferences in the US as well.)

Professional Training:

The IBE also provides professional training to those who want to turn their interest in healthy homes into a career. Many of their students are people already working in the building, design, housing, or health industries who want to supplement their knowledge so that they have a more wholistic view of both health and healthy homes. They offer a variety of levels of professional training each year through both online and face-to-face courses.

Where to Get Help:

Professional Assessment of Your Home or Office

In addition to the training courses they offer, the IBE can put you in contact with experienced building biologists to assess and consult on your home or office.

They can provide an analysis of your exposure to electromagnetic radiation and, depending upon your individual needs, the chemicals, moulds, and other toxins that could be affecting the indoor air quality of your building.

The links to these professionals are available on the 'Find an Expert' pages on the IBE website: *www.hbelc.org/findexpert.html*.

If there are no building biologists in your area, then seek out experienced electrical professionals who conduct EMR/electromagnetic surveys.

REFERENCES

Following are the pages where you'll find some of the references and sources used for research on this book:

During the years of my personal research into this subject, the two most fundamental and important sources of help and information have been:

George Carlo of the Science and Public Policy Institute (SPPI) in Washington DC, who ran what remains the world's largest research program addressing the dangers of cellular phones. It was funded by the wireless industry itself and overseen by the United States government. While the research found evidence of potential public health danger, there were strong economic and political pressures to suppress the information. Despite this, he went public with the danger warnings in the face of those pressures in 1999. In the ensuing decade of new research, those original warnings have so far been substantiated. The wealth of his experience has appeared in books, articles, and interviews on TV, radio, and magazines, and also through the CERSA training courses, which were run by the EMR University. (**www.secretsofchampions.org** and **www.safertech.com**)

Vicki Warren is the former executive director and program director of the Institute of Building Biology and Ecology (IBE) in the US. As a fully certified Building Biology and Environmental Consultant (BBEC) and Certified Electromagnetic Radiation Safety Advisor (CERSA), she now trains and consults through Wings of Eagles Healthy Living to help others regain and protect their health from exposure to electromagnetic radiation. Much of the information given here comes from Vicki's vast experience. (**www.wehliving.org/**)

My very first exposure to this subject, and information about its effects on health came from:

The International Institute of Building-Biology and Ecology (IBE) in the USA. The IBE runs professional and general interest courses on all aspects of how to make homes healthy, including in-depth information on all aspects of electromagnetic radiation. The starting point for my interest in, and research on, this subject was my training with the IBE in their:

> ➤ Building Biology Correspondence course

> ➤ Online Home Study courses

> ➤ Building Biology Professional Seminar Series

(There is a wealth of free information on their Web site: _www.hbelc.org_)

The knowledge passed on by the IBE trainers formed the initial impetus for the 'Hold The Phone' set of books. It was then built on by my own research, which included the research studies*, and additional information from the books, reports, and other sources listed on the following reference pages.

* The foundation for my work on these books was the research studies themselves. It was not felt practical to duplicate them here, as there are so many that it would have expanded the book's volume by an additional 50%.

The studies are listed in detail in the 'Research Studies' section of the companion book: **'Hold The Phone: Here's Why'.**

_"It takes two to speak truth.
One to speak, and another to hear."_

Henry David Thoreau

References (And Additional Reading Materials)

Books:

1.   Cell Phones: Invisible Hazards in the Wireless Age: An Insider's Alarming Discoveries about Cancer and Genetic Damage. George Carlo and Martin Schram. Basic Books, 2002.
2.   Cell Towers: Wireless Convenience? or Environmental Hazard? B Blake Levitt. Safe Goods, 2001.
3.   Public Health SOS: The Shadow Side of the Wireless Revolution. Camilla Rees and Magda Havas. Create Space Independent Publishing Platform, 2009.
4.   Would You Put Your Head in a Microwave Oven? Gerald Goldberg. AuthorHouse, 2006.
5.   Zapped: Why Your Cell Phone Shouldn't Be Your Alarm Clock, and 1268 Ways to Outsmart the Hazards of Electronic Pollution. Ann Louise Gittleman. HarperOne, 2011.
6.   The Force: Living Safely in a World of Electromagnetic Pollution. Lyn McLean. Scribe Publications, 2011.
7.   Cellular Telephone Russian Roulette. Robert C Kane. Vantage Pr, 2001.
8.   Cell Phones and the Dark Deception: Find Out What You're Not Being Told . . . And Why. Carleigh Cooper. Premier Advantage Publishing, 2009.
9.   Electromagnetic Fields: A Consumer's Guide to the Issues and How to Protect Ourselves. B Blake Levitt. Backinprint.com, 2007.
10.   The Powerwatch Handbook: Simple Ways to Make Your Environment Safer. Alasdair and Jean Philips. Piatkus Books, 2006.
11.   Warning: The electricity around you may be hazardous to your health. Ellen Sugarman. MiriamPress, 2004.
12.   The Electrical Sensitivity Handbook: How Electromagnetic Fields (EMFs) Are Making People Sick. Lucinda Grant. Weldon Publishing, 1995.
13.   Disconnect: The Truth About Cell Phone Radiation, What the Industry is Doing to Hide It, and How to Protect Your Family. Devra Davis. Plume, 2011.
14.   Dirty Electricity: Electrification and Diseases of Civilization. Sam Milham. iUniverse.com, 2010.
15.   The Invisible Disease: The Dangers of Environmental Illnesses Caused by Electromagnetic Fields and Chemical Emissions. Gunni Nordström. O Books, 2004.
16.   Electropollution: How to Protect Yourself Against It. Roger Coghill. Thorsons Publishing, 1990.
17.   Cross Currents: The Perils of Electropollution, the Promise of Electromedicine. Robert O Becker. Tarcher, 1990.
18.   iDisorder: Understanding Our Obsession with Technology and Overcoming Its Hold on Us. Larry Rosen. Palgrae Macmillan, 2012.

Articles, Letters, and Reports:

1.   Carlo G L. "Illusion and Escape: The Cell Phone Disease Quagmire. A Summary of American Legal Actions Regarding Mobile Phones and Health Effects"_http://www.naturalscience.org/fileadmin/portabledocuments/fact_sheet_no_01.pdf_
2.   Carlo G L. Letter to Maine Legislature, 24 March 2010. _http://www.scribd.com/doc/28894870/Letter-to-Maine-Legislature-Regarding-Warning-Label-Bill_
3.   Goldsworthy A. "Comments by Andrew Goldsworthy on Health Protection Agency Press Release entitled "Scientist probe laptops Wi-Fi Emissions." 20 Sept 2009 _http://www.radiationresearch.org/pdfs/20090926_hpa_wifi_ag_comments.pdf_
4.   Goldsworthy A. "Wi-Fi in Schools." _http://www.emfacts.com/2011/11/dr-andrew-goldsworthy-on-wi-fi-in-schools/_

5. Goldsworthy A. "Dr Andrew Goldsworthy Witness Statement April 2010." *http://www.mastsanity.org/health/research/292-dr-andrew-goldsworthy-witness-statement-april-2010.html*
6. Hemingway, P. "The risks to health from pulsed microwaves," An interview with Ingrid Dickenson, Homeopathy in practice, Spring 2006. *http://www.buergerwelle.de/assets/files/the_risk_to_health_from_pulsed_microwaves.pdf?cultureKey=&q=pdf/the_risk_to_health_from_pulsed_microwaves.pdf*
7. Hemingway, P. "What to do when electro-smog makes you sick." Homeopathy in practice, Summer 2006. *http://www.a-r-h.org/Publications/Journal/BackIssues.htm*
8. Ketcham, C. "Warning: Your Cell Phone May Be Hazardous to Your Health." GQ Magazine, Feburary 2010. *http://www.gq.com/cars-gear/gear-and-gadgets/201002/warning-cell-phone-radiation*
9. Khurana V. "Mobile Phones and Brain Tumours—A Public Health Concern." *http://www.brain-surgery.us/mobph.pdf*
10. Maisch, D. "Children and mobile phones—is there a health risk? The case for extra precautions". JACNEM, Vol. 22 No. 2; August 2003. *http://www.emfacts.com/papers/*
11. Maisch D. "Medical warnings needed on DECT cordless phone use." J. Aust. Coll. Nutr. & Env. Med. Vol. 25 No. 2 August 2006. *http://www.emfacts.com/papers/*
12. Maisch D. "Mobile Phone Use: It's time to take precautions." J. Aust. Coll. Nutr. & Env. Med. Vol. 20 No. 1 April 2001. *http://www.emfacts.com/papers/*
13. Morgan L Lloyd. "Cellphones and Brain Tumors: 15 Reasons for Concern. Science, Spin and the Truth Behind Interphone." L. Lloyd Morgan. *http://www.radiationresearch.org/pdfs/reasons_a4.pdf*
14. Phillips, A and J. Powerwatch. "Children & Mobile Phones: Parts 1–3." *http://www.powerwatch.org.uk/library/downloads/children-phones-1-use-2012-03.pdf http://www.powerwatch.org.uk/library/downloads/children-phones-2-advice-2012-03.pdf http://www.powerwatch.org.uk/library/downloads/children-phones-3-research-2012-03.pdf*
15. Philips, A and J. "Radiofrequency Protection for You and Your Family." *www.powerwatch.org.uk*
16. Philips, A and J. "Electrical Hypersensitivity, A Modern Illness." *www.powerwatch.org.uk*
17. Philips, A and J. "Radiofrequency EMF's and Health." *www.powerwatch.org.uk*
18. Philips, A and J. "Mobile Phones." *www.powerwatch.org.uk*
19. Starkey, Sarah H. "Living in a Wireless World." For the National Childbirth Trust. January 2010. *http://www.cavisoc.org.uk/National%20Childbirth%20Trust%20Jan%202010.pdf*
20. BioInitiative Working Group, Cindy Sage and David O. Carpenter, Editors. BioInitiative Report: A Rationale for a Biologically-based Public Exposure Standard for Electromagnetic Fields (ELF and RF) at www.bioinitiative.org August 31, 2007.
21. The Cell Phone Problem. "Cell Phones: Technology, Exposures, Health Effects."*http://www.ehhi.org/reports/cellphones/cell_phone_report_EHHI_Feb2012.pdf*
22. ICEMS—International Commission on Electromagnetic Safety. "Campaign for Safer Cell Phone Use." *http://www.icems.eu/public_education.htm*
23. "Joining the Dots: An Overview of Public Health Trends in 2007." The Australian Democrats. *http://www.democrats.org.au/docs/2007/Joining_the_Dots11.pdf*
24. Mobilewise. "Mobile phone health risks: the case for action to protect children." *http://www.mobilewise.org/wordpress/wpcontent/uploads/MobileWise_mobile_phone_health_risks_NEW.pdf*
25. "Safe Schools 2012: Medical and Scientific Experts Call For Safe Technologies in Schools." A document for schools. *http://wifiinschools.org.uk/resources/safeschools2012.pdf*
26. Gary Brown. "Wireless Devices, Standards, and Microwave Radiation in the Education Environment." October 2000. *http://www.getpurepower.ca/resources/WireleassDevices_GaryBrown.pdf*
27. "Wireless technologies and young people: A resource for schools." Wifiinschools.org.uk, October 2011. *http://wifiinschools.org.uk/resources/wireless+technologies+and+young+people+Oct2011.pdf*

YouTube:

1. BBC Panorama. Wi-Fi: A Warning Signal.
   Part 1: *http://www.youtube.com/watch?v=IuNaDj6VLHw*
   Part 2: *http://www.youtube.com/watch?v=yQGo0hesqIg&feature=relmfu*
   Part 3: *http://www.youtube.com/watch?v=VqnPtq4GbU*
2. *"Larry King Live*: Cell Phone Dangers." *http://www.youtube.com/watch?v=yKHg08f5_xo*
3. "Wi-Fi in Schools." *http://www.youtube.com/watch?v=IgLO9yR1JlQ*
4. "Wi-Fi in Schools is Proven Dangerous." *http://www.youtube.com/watch?v=KN7VetsCR2I*
5. "Cell Phone War." DVD. 2005. Filmmaker Klaus Scheidsteger.
6. "Public Exposure: DNA, Democracy and the 'Wireless Revolution.'" Co-produced by EON, The Ecological Options Network and the Council on Wireless Technology Impacts.
7. "Is it safe or not?" Johansson, O: (In 15 parts)
   Part 1: *http://www.youtube.com/watch?v=eS7YIZ1x0r8*
8. "Dangers of cell phone wi-fi radiation". Carlo, G L.
   Part 1: *http://www.youtube.com/watch?v=kofG4W74tIE*.
   Part 2: *http://www.youtube.com/watch?v=Urzibz5_CyQ*.
   Part 3: *http://www.youtube.com/watch?v=YHVaK0Ih08c*
9. "Wi-Fi in schools proven dangerous." *http://www.youtube.com/watch?v=KN7VetsCR2I& lr=1&uid=qhEjmO5kntxIoouAOYm16Q*
10. Smart Meters and EMR: The Health Crisis of Our Time—Dr Dietrich Klinghardt. *http:// www.youtube.com/watch?v=b_wxM6IAFII*

Radio Interviews:

1. "Your Own Health and Fitness."   Radio Show with Jeffry Fawcett and Layna Berman. Interview: "Health Considerations for the Digital Revolution," with B Blake Levitt. (4.24.2012)
2. "Your Own Health and Fitness."   Radio Show with Jeffry Fawcett and Layna Berman. Interview: "Industry Censored Cell Phone Science," with Devra Davis. (10.5.2010)
3. "Your Own Health and Fitness."   Radio Show with Jeffry Fawcett and Layna Berman. Interview: "Wireless Risks in the Mainstream," with Christopher Ketcham and Michael Segell. (2.9.2010)
4. "Your Own Health and Fitness."   Radio Show with Jeffry Fawcett and Layna Berman. Interview: "Wireless Technology Health News," with Cindy Sage. (10.27.2009)
5. "Your Own Health and Fitness."   Radio Show with Jeffry Fawcett and Layna Berman. Interview: "Alternatives to Wireless Broadband," with Doug Loranger and Sally Hampton.
6. "Your Own Health and Fitness."   Radio Show with Jeffry Fawcett and Layna Berman. Interview: "Secondhand Cell Phone Radiation," with Cindy Sage. (10.28.2008)
7. "Your Own Health and Fitness."   Radio Show with Jeffry Fawcett and Layna Berman. Interview: "Hypersensitivity, a discussion." (4.1.2008)
8. "Your Own Health and Fitness."   Radio Show with Jeffry Fawcett and Layna Berman. Interview:
9. "Wi-Max, the Next Wireless Exposure," with Libby Kelley. (12.4.2007)
10. "Your Own Health and Fitness."   Radio Show with Jeffry Fawcett and Layna Berman. Interview:
11. "The Science of RFR Health Risks," with Olle Johanssen. (4.25.2006)
12. "Your Own Health and Fitness."   Radio Show with Jeffry Fawcett and Layna Berman. Interview: "Wireless Public Health Crisis," with B Blake Levitt, Jan Newton and Doug Loranger. (2.7.2006)

Documentary DVDs:

1. Full Signal: The Hidden Cost of Cellphones. Directed by Talal Jabari. *www.fullsignalmovie. com*
2. Cell Phone War. Filmmaker Klaus Scheidsteger. DVD of documentary aired on French TV, 2005.
3. Public Exposure: DNA, Democracy and the Wireless Revolution. Co-produced by EON, The Ecological Options Network and the Council on Wireless Technology Impacts
4. Resonance: Beings of Frequency. A James Russell film; Flat Frog Productions, 2012. *www.flatfrogfilms.com/resonance-documentary/*

References for the Experts' Quotes:

1. BioInitiative Working Group, Cindy Sage and David O Carpenter, Editors. BioInitiative Report: A Rationale for a Biologically-based Public Exposure Standard for Electromagnetic Fields (ELF and RF) at www.bioinitiative.org. August 31, 2007.
2. Siegal Sadetzki in: Martin Beckford. "Department of Health under pressure to increase precautions over children's mobile phone use." Daily Telegraph, 24 October 2009. *http://www.telegraph.co.uk/health/healthnews/6417245/Department-of-Health-under-pressure-to-increase-precautions-over-childrens-mobile-phone-use.html*
3. Salford, L. "Non-thermal effects of EMF upon the mammalian brain,' a presentation made an international conference entitled "The Precautionary EMF Approach: Rationale, Legislation and Implementation," convened by the International Commission for Electromagnetic Safety and hosted by the City of Benevento, Italy, in February 2006. *http://www.icems.eu/docs/Salford.pdf*
4. WHO / IARC. "IARC Classifies Radiofrequency Electromagnetic Fields as Possibly Carcinogenic to Humans." *http://www.iarc.fr/en/media-centre/pr/2011/pdfs/pr208_E.pdf*
5. Franz Adlkofer. "German radiation protection offside. Pandora: Foundation for Independent Research, 2011.*http://www.pandora-foundation.eu/downloads/pandora_news_comment-on-iarc-decision-2011.pdf*
6. Alasdair Philips in: "Be Aware: These Cell Phones Can Emit 28 Times More Radiation." Mercola.com: *http://articles.mercola.com/sites/articles/archive/2011/06/18/finally-experts-admit-cellphones-are-a-carcinogen.aspx*
7. Joel Moskowitz. "IARC Classifies Radiofrequency Electromagnetic Fields as Possibly Carcinogenic to Humans." Electromagnetic Health. *http://electromagnetichealth.org/electromagnetic-health-blog/iarc-rf-carc/*
8. Cindy Sage in: "Public Exposure: DNA, Democracy and the Wireless Revolution." DVD. EON, The Ecological Options Network and the Council on Wireless Technology Impacts. 2000.
9. Alasdair Philips in: Susie Boniface, Adrian Butler. "Health study links mobile phone use to four kinds of cancer." Mirror, October 25, 2009. *http://www.mirror.co.uk/news/top-stories/2009/10/25/new-cancer-link-to-mobiles-115875-21771409/#*
10. Guiliani L, Soffritti M. Non-Thermal effects and mechanisms of interaction between electromagnetic fields and living matter. Eur. J. Oncol. Library, vol. 5. 2010.
11. George Carlo in: "Cell Phone War." Filmmaker Klaus Scheidsteger. DVD of documentary aired on French TV, 2005.
12. Tara Parker-Pope. "Experts Revive Debate Over Cellphones and Cancer." New York Times. June 3, 2008. *http://www.nytimes.com/2008/06/03/health/03well.html?_r=1*
13. Bengt Arnetz in: "Mobiles linked to disturbed sleep." BBC News. January 21, 2008. *http://news.bbc.co.uk/2/hi/health/7199659.stm*
14. Ross Adey in: "Worry about your Wireless?" 20/20-with Barbara Walters: ABC News. May 26, 2000. *http://www.sarshield.com/news/wirelessworry2020.html*
15. Levis AG et al. Mobile phones and head tumours: it is time to read and highlight data in a proper way. Epidemiol Prev. 2011 May-Aug;35(3-4):188-99.
16. Sato Y et al. A case-case study of mobile phone use and acoustic neuroma risk in Japan. Bioelectromagnetics 32(2):85–93 February, 2011. *http://www.emf-portal.org/viewer.php?l=e&aid=18715*

17. Cindy Sage. "Plain Talk About Cell Phone Safety." September 22, 2009. *http:// emfsafetynetwork.org/wp-content/uploads/2009/11/Plain-Talk-on-Cell-Phones1.pdf*
18. Lawrence Challis in: Martin Beckford. "Department of Health under pressure to increase precautions over children's mobile phone use." Daily Telegraph. October 24, 2009. *http://www.telegraph.co.uk/health/healthnews/6417245/Department-of-Health-under-pressure-to-increase-precautions-over-childrens-mobile-phone-use.html*
19. Vicki Warren. "Never use your cell phone in a plane, train, or metal building—Here's why." January 7, 2010. Mercola.com. *http://emf.mercola.com/sites/emf/archive/2010/01/07/ Never-Use-Your-Cell-Phone-in-a-Plain-Train-or-Metal-Building-Heres-Why.aspx*
20. Kjell Hansson Mild in: Mi Kai Lee. "Cell phone health concerns continue to spread." Columbia Valley News. March 10, 2009. *http://weepnews.blogspot.com.au/2009/03/cell-phone-health-concerns-continue-to.html*
21. Orjan Hallberg in: "Quotations from Scientists, Physicians and others." Radiation research: *http://archive.radiationresearch.org/pdfs/reasons_quotes.pdf*
22. Vicki Warren. "Never use your cell phone in a plane, train, or metal building—Here's why." January 7, 2010. Mercola.com. *http://emf.mercola.com/sites/emf/archive/2010/01/07/ Never-Use-Your-Cell-Phone-in-a-Plain-Train-or-Metal-Building-Heres-Why.aspx*
23. David Strayer in: "Cell phone users drive like old folks." University of Utah, News Center. February 1, 2005. *www.unews.utah.edu/p/?r=022106-52*
24. Alvaro Augusto A de Salles in: Quotations from Scientists, Physicians and others." Radiation research. *http://archive.radiationresearch.org/pdfs/reasons_quotes.pdf*.
25. Sage and Associates. "What to tell your employer about cell phones and PDA's in the workplace—Neurological Effects of Wireless Technologies. Talking Points on Cell Phones and Health Risks." September 2009. *www.emrpolicy.org/files/responsible_corporate_policy.pdf*
26. Neil Cherry in: "Health Effects from Cell Phone Tower Radiation". Karen J Rogers. 2002. *http://www.docstoc.com/docs/13267006/Health-Effects-from-Cell-Phone-Tower-Radiation*
27. George Carlo in: "Cell Phone War." Filmmaker Klaus Scheidsteger. DVD of documentary aired on French TV, 2005.
28. Martin Blank. Section 7: "Evidence for Stress Response." BioInitiative Report: A Rationale for a Biologically-based Public Exposure Standard for Electromagnetic Fields (ELF and RF) at www.bioinitiative.org. August 31, 2007.
29. Email to mailing list, Microwave News, August 16 2009.
30. Alasdair Philips in: Susie Boniface, Adrian Butler. "Health study links mobile phone use to four kinds of cancer." Mirror. October 25, 2009. *http://www.mirror.co.uk/news/top-stories/2009/10/25/new-cancer-link-to-mobiles-115875-21771409/#*
31. Andrew Goldsworthy. "Dr Goldsworthy responds to HPA's 'no risk' Wi-Fi Press Release: Press Release by the Health Protection Agency on 15th Sept 2009 entitled 'Scientist probe laptops Wi-Fi Emissions.'" Mast Sanity, September 20, 2009. *http://www.mastsanity.org/ index.php?option=com_content&task=view&id=279&Itemid=1*
32. "Global mobile statistics 2012 Part C: Mobile marketing, advertising and messaging." mobiThinking, June 2012. *http://mobithinking.com/mobile-marketing-tools/latest-mobile-stats/c*
33. Michael Lerner in: The President's Cancer Panel. Annual Report 2008–2009. *http:// deainfo.nci.nih.gov/advisory/pcp/pcp08-09rpt/PCP_Report_08-09_508.pdf*
34. Olga Naidenko in: Bryan Walsh. "Cell Phone Radiation Risks: Why the Jury's Still Out." Time, September 22, 2009. *http://www.time.com/time/health/article/0,8599,1925152,00. html*
35. Johansson, O. "Disturbance of the immune system by electromagnetic fields—A potentially underlying cause for cellular damage and tissue repair reduction which could lead to disease and impairment." Pathophysiology 2009 Aug;16(2–3):157–77. *http://www.regjeringen.no/ pages/2211863/Thomas%20J%20Middelthon%20vedlegg.pdf*
36. "Cell Phone War." Filmmaker Klaus Scheidsteger. DVD of documentary aired on French TV, 2005.
37. Paul J Rosch. "Expressions of Concern from Scientists, Physicians, Health Policy Experts and Others." Electromagnetic Health. *http://electromagnetichealth.org/quotes-from-experts/*

38. George Carlo. "Illusion and Escape: The Cell Phone Disease Quagmire. A Summary of American Legal Actions Regarding Mobile Phones and Health Effects." The American Trial Lawyer. Fall 2008. *http://www.naturalscience.org/fileadmin/portabledocuments/ fact_sheet_no_01.pdf*
39. Personal correspondence between Vicki Warren and the author, June 23, 2010.
40. Ross Adey in: David Kirkpatrick. Interview with Ross Adey. Fortune Magazine, October 9, 2000.
41. Bengt Arnetz in: "Mobiles linked to insomnia." The Sydney Morning Herald. January 22, 2008. *http://www.smh.com.au/news/technology/mobiles-linked-to-insomnia/2008/01/22/1200764222494.html*
42. Geoffrey Lean. "Mobile phone radiation wrecks your sleep. Phone makers own scientists discover that bedtime use can lead to headaches, confusion and depression." The Independent, January 20, 2008. *http://www.independent.co.uk/life-style/health-and-families/ health-news/mobile-phone-radiation-wrecks-your-sleep-771262.html*
43. Dimitris Panagopulos. "Electromagnetic Interaction between Environmental Fields and Living Systems Determines Health and Well-Being" in "Electromagnetic Fields: Principles, Engineering Applications and Biophysical Effects" 2013, Hauppauge, New York Nova Science Publishers
44. Neil Cherry. "Possible Biological and Health Effects of Radio Frequency Electromagnetic Fields." University of Vienna Workshop: Summary Report. October 1998.
45. Andrew Goldsworthy. "Dr Goldsworthy responds to HPA's 'no risk' Wi-Fi Press Release: Press Release by the Health Protection Agency on 15th Sept 2009 entitled 'Scientist probe laptops Wi-Fi Emissions.'" Mast Sanity, September 20, 2009. *http://www.mastsanity.org/ index.php?option=com_content&task=view&id=279&Itemid=1*
46. Larry D Rosen. iDisorder: Understanding our obsession with technology and overcoming its hold on us. (Palgrave Macmillan. 2012.) Page 49.
47. Safe Wireless Initiative. Medical Alert. "Aggravated Symptom Relapses Reported after Use of Widely-Available EMR Protection Products." *http://www.etudesetvie.be/files/ images/EMR-IP/Medicalalert-En.pdf*
48. Levi Schachter in: "Mobile Phones could be damaging your eyesight." Powerwatch. August 8, 2005. *http://www.powerwatch.org.uk/news/20050808_eyesight.asp*
49. Paul J Rosch. "Expressions of Concern from Scientists, Physicians, Health Policy Experts and Others." Electromagnetic Health. *http://electromagnetichealth.org/quotes-from-experts/*
50. Valerie Strauss. "Social media addiction: Worse than you think." The Washington Post, April 28, 2010. *http://voices.washingtonpost.com/answer-sheet/research/social-media-addiction-study-w.html*
51. Larry D Rosen. iDisorder: Understanding our obsession with technology and overcoming its hold on us. (Palgrave Macmillan. 2012.) Page 107.
52. "Mobile phone safety: The real truth about the hazards, told by independent scientists." PSRAST: Physicians and Scientists for Responsible Application of Science & Technology. *http://www.psrast.org/mobileng/mobilstarteng.htm#junk*
53. "Cellphones and Brain Tumors: 15 Reasons for Concern, Science, Spin and the Truth Behind Interphone." L Lloyd Morgan, primary author. International EMF Collaborative. August 25, 2009. *http://www.radiationresearch.org/pdfs/reasons_us.pdf*
54. ibid.
55. Camilla Rees. "FCC Cell Phone Safety Guidelines Underestimate Harmful Radiation Absorbed by Children and Small Adults, Says New Analysis." EMFacts Consultancy. October 17, 2011. *http://www.emfacts.com/2011/10/fcc-cell-phone-safety-guidelines-underestimate-harmful-radiation-absorbed-by-children-and-small-adults-says-new-analysis/*
56. The President's Cancer Panel. Annual Report 2008-2009 *http://deainfo.nci.nih.gov/ advisory/pcp/pcp08-09rpt/PCP_Report_08-09_508.pdf*
57. George Carlo. "Illusion and Escape: The Cell Phone Disease Quagmire. A Summary of American Legal Actions Regarding Mobile Phones and Health Effects." The American Trial Lawyer. Fall 2008. *http://www.naturalscience.org/fileadmin/portabledocuments/ fact_sheet_no_01.pdf*
58. Anne Campbell. "Cordless home phones sparks radiation fear." Mail Online, February 6, 2006. *http://www.dailymail.co.uk/health/article-376279/Cordless-home-phones-sparks-radiation-fear.html#ixzz0Q5vvMgEY*

59. Lennart Hardell in: "BioInitiative Report 2007: Press Release." A summary of findings and quotes from authors. *http://www.bioinitiative.org/freeaccess/press_release/index.htm*
60. "DECT—The Radiation Source at Home : Cordless Phones radiate unnecessarily." German Federal Agency for Radiation Protection. (Bundesamt für Strahlenschutz—BfS). Press Release. January 31, 2006. *http://www.emfacts.com/2006/02/offical-warning-on-dect-phones/*
61. Olle Johansson in: Sarah Benson. "Do adverse health trends correlate with research into Electromagnetic Radiation (EMR)? An overview of adverse public health trends from 1996–2009." NZine, October 8, 2009. *http://www.nzine.co.nz/features/electromagnetic_radiation.html*
62. Haumann T and Sierck P. "Non-stop Pulsed 2.4 GHz Radiation Inside US Homes." Presented at 2nd International Workshop on Biological Effects of Electromagnetic Fields. 7–11 October 2002. *http://bemri.org/publications/cat_view/2-publications/5-biological-effects-of-non-ionizing-radiation/47-dect.html?limit=20&limitstart=0&order=date&dir=ASC*
63. Gerd Oberfeld. "Electropollution in our environment." Lecture given at the Annual Meeting on behalf of Irish Doctors Environmental Association (IDEA), University of Cork, Ireland, February 2009. *www.ideaireland.org/electromagnetic_pollution_oberfeld_2009.pdf*
64. Alasdair Philips and Jean Philips. The Power Watch Handbook. (London: Piatkus Books Ltd, 2006) 294.
65. Alasdair Philips in: Anne Campbell. "Cordless home phones sparks radiation fear." Mail Online, February 6, 2006. *http://www.dailymail.co.uk/health/article-376279/Cordless-home-phones-sparks-radiation-fear.html#ixzz0Q5vvMgEY*
66. Don Maisch. "Medical warnings needed on DECT cordless phone and newer DECT baby monitors." J. Aust. Coll. Nutr. & Env. Med. Vol. 25 No. 2 August 2006
67. "A phone mast in your home?" Wired Child. *http://wiredchild.org/sciencealias/43-what-the-science-tells-us/67-what-the-science-tells-us-wireless-products.html*
68. Lukas Margaritis in: "Greek Researchers Show Crucial Regions of the Brain Related to Learning, Memory, Alzheimer's Impacted by Whole Body EMF Exposure in Animals". Electromagnetic Health. January 25, 2012. *www.electromagnetichealth.org/electromagnetic-health-blog/mice-proteome/*
69. Cindy Sage. Section 1: Public Summary for the Public. BioInitiative Working Group, Cindy Sage and David O. Carpenter, Editors. BioInitiative Report: A Rationale for a Biologically-based Public Exposure Standard for Electromagnetic Fields (ELF and RF) at www.bioinitiative.org. August 31, 2007.
70. Andrew Goldsworthy in: Walter Graham. "Dangers of Wi-Fi in schools." Voice: the union of education professionals. *http://www.voicetheunion.org.uk/index.cfm?cid=704*
71. Geoffrey Lean. "Germany warns citizens to avoid using Wi-Fi." The Independent, September 9, 2007. *http://www.independent.co.uk/environment/green-living/germany-warns-citizens-to-avoid-using-wifi-401845.html*
72. BioInitiative Working Group, Cindy Sage and David O. Carpenter, Editors. BioInitiative Report: A Rationale for a Biologically-based Public Exposure Standard for Electromagnetic Fields (ELF and RF) at www.bioinitiative.org. August 31, 2007.
73. "CTIA Survey Show More Wireless Devices than Americans." CTIA The Wireless Association. October 11, 2011. *http://blog.ctia.org/2011/10/11/ctia-survey-show-more-wireless-devices-than-americans/*
74. Paul J Rosch. "Expressions of Concern from Scientists, Physicians, Health Policy Experts and Others." Electromagnetic Health. *http://electromagnetichealth.org/quotes-from-experts/*
75. "Presentation of Prof Dominique Belpomme at 8th National Congress on Electrosmog, Berne 2011." Weep News, June 11, 2011. *http://weepnews.blogspot.com/2011/06/presentation-of-prof-dominique-belpomme.html*
76. "Scientists Urge Halt of Wireless Rollout and Call for New Safety Standards: Warning Issued on Risks to Children and Pregnant Women." Press Release from the Karolinska Institute, Department of Neuroscience, Stockholm, Sweden, February 3, 2011. *http://www.scribd.com/doc/48148346/Karolinska-Institute-Press-Release*
77. "Libraries switch off Wi-Fi internet." The Connexion, June 4, 2008. *http://www.connexionfrance.com/news_articles.php?id=173*
78. BioInitiative Working Group, Cindy Sage and David O Carpenter, Editors. BioInitiative Report: A Rationale for a Biologically-based Public Exposure Standard for Electromagnetic Fields (ELF and RF) at www.bioinitiative.org. August 31, 2007.

79. Andrew Goldsworthy. "Dr Goldsworthy responds to HPA's 'no risk' Wi-Fi Press Release: Press Release by the Health Protection Agency on 15th Sept 2009 entitled 'Scientist probe laptops Wi-Fi Emissions.'" Mast Sanity, September 20, 2009. *http://www.mastsanity.org/index.php?option=com_content&task=view&id=279&Itemid=1*

80. B Blake Levitt. "Expressions of Concern from Scientists, Physicians, Health Policy Experts and Others." Electromagnetic Health. *http://electromagnetichealth.org/quotes-from-experts/*

81. Lukas Margaritis in: "Scientists Urge Halt of Wireless Rollout and Call for New Safety Standards: Warning Issued on Risks to Children and Pregnant Women." Press Release from the Karolinska Institute, Department of Neuroscience, Stockholm, Sweden, February 3, 2011. *http://www.scribd.com/doc/48148346/Karolinska-Institute-Press-Release*

82. Lloyd Morgan in: Seth Koenig. "Scientists at Portland seminar liken cell phones to smoking." BDN Maine: Health, October 17, 2011. *http://bangordailynews.com/2011/10/17/health/scientists-at-portland-seminar-liken-cellphones-to-smoking/?ref=latest*

83. Ian Gibson in: "Wi-Fi: A Warning Signal." Panorama, BBC One, May 21, 2007. *http://news.bbc.co.uk/2/hi/programmes/panorama/6683969.stm*

84. Nicholas Negroponte. "Being Wireless: Why Wi-Fi 'lily pads and frogs' will transform the future of telecom. Wired. *http://www.wired.com/wired/archive/10.10/wireless_pr.html*

85. Ibid.

86. Andrew Goldsworthy. "Dr Goldsworthy responds to HPA's 'no risk' Wi-Fi Press Release: Press Release by the Health Protection Agency on 15th Sept 2009 entitled 'Scientist probe laptops Wi-Fi Emissions.'" Mast Sanity, September 20, 2009. *http://www.mastsanity.org/index.php?option=com_content&task=view&id=279&Itemid=1*

87. Avendano C et al. "Laptop Expositions affect motility and induce DNA fragmentation in Human spermatozoa in vitro by a non-thermal effect: A preliminary report." Presented at 2010 Annual ASRM meeting. *http://www.emfacts.com/weblog/?p=1358*

88. BioInitiative Working Group, Cindy Sage and David O Carpenter, Editors. BioInitiative Report: A Rationale for a Biologically-based Public Exposure Standard for Electromagnetic Fields (ELF and RF) at www.bioinitiative.org. August 31, 2007.

89. "CTIA Survey Show More Wireless Devices than Americans." CTIA The Wireless Association. October 11, 2011. *http://blog.ctia.org/2011/10/11/ctia-survey-show-more-wireless-devices-than-americans/*

90. Sarah J Starkey in: "Scientists around the world have been speaking out: The Bio-Initiative Report. Other scientists have commented on the evidence . . ." Wired Child. *http://wiredchild.org/sciencealias/43-what-the-science-tells-us/65-what-scientists-are-saying.html*

91. Arnetz B et al. "The Effects of 884 MHz GSM Wireless Communication Signals on Self-reported Symptom and Sleep (EEG) - An Experimental Provocation Study." 2007. PIERS Online 3(7):1148–1150. *http://www.piers.org/piersonline/pdf/Vol3No7Page1148to1150.pdf*

92. Martin Blank. BioInitiative Report Press Release: BioInitiative Working Group, Cindy Sage and David O Carpenter, Editors. BioInitiative Report: A Rationale for a Biologically-based Public Exposure Standard for Electromagnetic Fields (ELF and RF) at www.bioinitiative.org. August 31, 2007.

93. George Carlo in: Albert Roman. "Cell Phones, the New Cigarettes." The Epoch Times, February 25, 2009. *http://www.theepochtimes.com/n2/content/view/12653/*

94. Gerald Hyland in: "What a Cell Phone Can Do to a Child's Brain in Just Two Minutes." The Mirror, December 26, 2001. *http://www.rawfoodinfo.com/articles/art_cellphchild.html*

95. Panagopoulos DJ, Johansson O, Carlo GL (2013) Evaluation of Specific Absorption Rate as a Dosimetric Quantity for Electromagnetic Fields Bioeffects. PLoS ONE 8(6): e62663.

96. Gandhi OP et al. Exposure limits: the underestimation of absorbed cell phone radiation, especially in children. Electromagn Biol Med. 2012 Mar;31(1):34-51

97. Children's use of mobile phones: An international comparison 2011. GSMA, NTT DOCOMO special report, 2011, November 22. *www.gsma.com/publicpolicy/childrens-use-of-mobile-phones-an-international-comparison-executive-summary-spanish-november-2011-japan-india-paraguay-and-egypt* *http://www.guardian.co.uk/media/2001/jun/29/newmedia.schools*

98. Sage and Associates. "What to tell your employer about cell phones and PDA's in the workplace—Neurological Effects of Wireless Technologies. Talking Points on Cell Phones and Health Risks." September 2009. *www.emrpolicy.org/files/responsible_corporate_policy.pdf*

99. "Children and Mobile Phones: The Health of the Following Generations is in Danger." Russian National Committee on Non-Ionizing Radiation Protection, Moscow, Russia. 14th April 2008. www.radiationresearch.org/pdfs/rncnirp_children.pdf

100. Larry D Rosen. iDisorder: Understanding our obsession with technology and overcoming its hold on us. (Palgrave Macmillan. 2012.) Page 104.

101. Mariea T, Carlo GL. Wireless Radiation in the Etiology and Treatment of Autism: Clinical Observations

102. and Mechanisms. J Aust Col. Nutr & Env Med 2007 August, Vol. 26 (2) 3–7.

103. Geoffrey Lean. "Warning: Using a mobile phone while pregnant can seriously damage the health of your baby." The Independent, May 18, 2008. http://www.independent.co.uk/life-style/health-and-families/health-news/warning-using-a-mobile-phone-while-pregnant-can-seriously-damage-your-baby-830352.html

104. Nina Lakhani. "A close call: Why the jury is still out on mobile phones." The Independent, April, 24 2012. http://www.independent.co.uk/life-style/gadgets-and-tech/news/a-close-call-why-the-jury-is-still-out-on-mobile-phones-7670543.html

105. Yuri Grigoriev in: "Important New Russian Research on Cell Phone Radiation's Effect on Cognitive and Other Functions in Children." Electromagnetic Health. April 11, 2011. http://electromagnetichealth.org/electromagnetic-health-blog/russian-res-children-emf/

106. Geoffrey Lean. "Mobile phone use 'raises children's risk of brain cancer fivefold.'" The Independent, September 21, 2008. http://www.independent.co.uk/news/science/mobile-phone-use-raises-childrens-risk-of-brain-cancer-fivefold-937005.html

107. "Dr Carlo on Children and Health Damage from Mobile Phones." Mast Sanity. http://www.mastsanity.org/home/2/280-dr-george-carlo-on-children-and-health-damage-from-mobile-phones.html

108. Erik Huber in: Alasdair Philips and Jean Philips. "Children and Mobile Phones 3: The Research." Powerwatch. http://www.powerwatch.org.uk/library/downloads/children-phones-3-research-2012-03.pdf

109. Chris Woollams in: "Cellphones and Brain Tumors: 15 Reasons for Concern, Science, Spin and the Truth Behind Interphone. L Lloyd Morgan, primary author. International EMF Collaborative. August 25, 2009. http://www.radiationresearch.org/pdfs/reasons_us.pdf

110. Paul J Rosch in: "Expressions of Concern from Scientists, Physicians, Health Policy Experts and Others." Electromagnetic Health. http://electromagnetichealth.org/quotes-from-experts/

111. Michael Kundi. "More Reasons Children May Be at Risk." Microwave News, Vol. 22, No. 4, p 13, July/ August 2002.

112. Vini Khurana in: "Is there a link between cell phones and cancer?" Transcript: Larry King Live, CNN, May 27, 2008. http://transcripts.cnn.com/TRANSCRIPTS/0805/27/lkl.01.html

113. Gene Barnett in: Julie A Evans. "The Cell Tolls for Thee: The truth about the cell-phone-cancer link, and what it means for you and your kids." Best Life, August 2008. http://www.giadownloads.com/pdf/MSN_Health_Fitness.pdf

114. Om Gandhi in: Alasdair Philips and Jean Philips. "Children and Mobile Phones 3: The Research Findings." Powerwatch. http://www.powerwatch.org.uk/library/downloads/children-phones-3-research-2012-03.pdf

115. Abramson MJ et al. Mobile telephone use is associated with changes in cognitive function in young adolescents. Bioelectromagnetics. 2009 Dec;30(8):678-86. http://www.ncbi.nlm.nih.gov/pubmed/19644978

116. Annie Sasco in: Nina Lakhani . "A close call: Why the jury is still out on mobile phones." The Independent, April, 24 2012. http://www.independent.co.uk/life-style/gadgets-and-tech/news/a-close-call-why-the-jury-is-still-out-on-mobile-phones-7670543.html

117. L Lloyd Morgan in: "Cellphones and Brain Tumors: 15 Reasons for Concern, Science, Spin and the Truth Behind Interphone." L Lloyd Morgan, primary author. International EMF Collaborative. August 25, 2009. http://www.radiationresearch.org/pdfs/reasons_us.pdf

118. Geoffrey Lean. "Radiation from baby monitors poses risk." The Irish Independent, May 21, 2007. http://www.independent.ie/lifestyle/parenting/radiation-from-baby-monitors-poses-risk-680514.html
119. Don Maisch. "Medical warnings needed on DECT cordless phone and newer DECT baby monitors." J. Aust. Coll. Nutr. & Env. Med. Vol. 25 No. 2 August 2006 (accepted for publication).
120. Alasdair Philips, Jean Philips. "Digital Cordless Baby Monitors—Our Experiences." Powerwatch. http://www.powerwatch.org.uk/news/20060222_baby_monitors.asp
121. Geoffrey Lean. "Radiation from baby monitors poses risk." The Irish Independent, May 21, 2007. http://www.independent.ie/lifestyle/parenting/radiation-from-baby-monitors-poses-risk-680514.html
122. Paul J Rosch in: "Expressions of Concern from Scientists, Physicians, Health Policy Experts and Others." Electromagnetic Health. http://electromagnetichealth.org/quotes-from-experts/
123. Yuri Grigoriev in: "Scientists Urge Halt of Wireless Rollout and Call for New Safety Standards: Warning Issued on Risks to Children and Pregnant Women." Press Release from the Karolinska Institute, Department of Neuroscience, Stockholm, Sweden, February 3, 2011. http://www.scribd.com/doc/48148346/Karolinska-Institute-Press-Release
124. Sarah J Starkey. "Living in a wireless world." For the National Childbirth Trust. January 2010. http://www.cavisoc.org.uk/National%20Childbirth%20Trust%20Jan%202010.pdf
125. Elizabeth Barris in: Albert Roman. "Cell Phones, the New Cigarettes." The Epoch Times, February 25, 2009. http://www.theepochtimes.com/n2/content/view/12653/
126. Alasdair Philips in: Nic Fleming. "Warning on Wi-Fi health risk to Children." The Telegraph, April 28, 2007. http://www.telegraph.co.uk/news/uknews/1549944/Warning-on-wi-fi-health-risk-to-children.html
127. Rory Watson. "Radiation fears prompt possible restrictions on wi-fi and mobile phone use in schools." British Medical Journal, July 26, 2011. http://www.bmj.com/content/342/bmj.d3428.extract
128. Elizabeth Barris in: Albert Roman. "Cell Phones, the New Cigarettes." The Epoch Times, February 25, 2009. http://www.theepochtimes.com/n2/content/view/12653/
129. Thomas Rau in: Camilla Rees. "Medical Director of Switzerland's Paracelsus Clinic Takes Stand on Hazards of Electromagnetic Pollution—'Electromagnetic Load' a Hidden Factor in Many Illnesses." Electromagnetic Health. February 10, 2009. http://electromagnetichealth.org/electromagnetic-health-blog/medical-director-of-switzerland/
130. Gerd Oberfeld in: "Wi-Fi: A Warning Signal." Panorama, BBC One, May 21, 2007. http://news.bbc.co.uk/2/hi/programmes/panorama/6683969.stm
131. Olle Johansson. "WLAN in Schools." Letter in reply to Concerned Parent, October 6, 2005. http://www.powerwatch.org.uk/pdfs/20070723_wifi_olle.pdf
132. David O Carpenter in: "Expressions of Concern from Scientists, Physicians, Health Policy Experts and Others." Electromagnetic Health. http://electromagnetichealth.org/quotes-from-experts/
133. "Dr Andrew Goldsworthy on Wi-Fi in Schools." EMFacts Consultancy, November 9, 2011. http://www.emfacts.com/2011/11/dr-andrew-goldsworthy-on-wi-fi-in-schools/
134. Geoffrey Lean. "Wi-Fi: Children at risk from 'electronic smog.'" The Independent, April 22, 2007. http://www.independent.co.uk/life-style/health-and-families/health-news/wifi-children-at-risk-from-electronic-smog-445725.html
135. Devra Lee Davis in: "Health Canada has little to say about cellphone risks for kids." CBCnews.ca. January 22, 2009. http://www.cbc.ca/news/health/story/2009/01/22/cellphone-children.html
136. "Understanding the Science. "Wired Child. www.wiredchild.org/sciencealias.html
137. Carl Hilliard in: "Cell Phone War." Filmmaker Klaus Scheidsteger. DVD of documentary aired on French TV, 2005.

Cell Phones

1. Hondou T et al. Passive Exposure to Mobile Phones: Enhancement of Intensity by Reflection. *J. Phys. Soc. Jpn.* 75 (2006) 084801. *http://jpsj.ipap.jp/link?JPSJ/75/084801/*
2. Hondou T. Rising Level of Public Exposure to Mobile Phones: Accumulation through Additivity and Reflectivity. *J. Phys. Soc. Jpn.* 71 (2002) pp. 432–435. *http://jpsj.ipap.jp/link?JPSJ/71/432/*
3. Arthur Firstenberg. "The Largest Biological Experiment Ever." *Sun Monthly*, January 1, 2006. *www.mindfully.org/Technology/2006/Firstenberg-EMF-Experiment1jan06.htm*

4. Janet Raloff. "Cell phones: Precautions Recommended." *Science News*, September 16, 2009. *http://www.sciencenews.org/view/generic/id/47430/title/Science_%2B_the_Public_Cell_phones_Precautions_recommended*
5. The Human Project interview with Olle Johansson. "Mobile Phone Radiation: Is it safe or not? That is the question?" *http://www.bevolution.dk/pdf/MobilePhoneRadiationIsitsafeornot.pdf*
6. Alasdair Philips and Jean Philips. "Young children's use of mobile phones soars in the UK." Powerwatch, 11.1.2010. *http://www.powerwatch.org.uk/news/20100111_mobile_phones_kids.asp*
7. Sage C, Johansson O, Sage SA. Personal digital assistant (PDA) cell phone units produce elevated extremely-low frequency electromagnetic field emissions. *Bioelectromagnetics*. 2007 Jul;28(5):386-92. *http://www.buergerwelle.de/pdf/sage_pda_bems_on_line.pdf*
8. Cindy Sage. "Personal Digital Assistant (PDA) Cell Phone Units Produce Elevated Extremely-Low Frequency Electromagnetic Field Emissions." *Omega News*, March 17, 2007. *http://omega.twoday.net/stories/3446388/*
9. George Carlo. "Letter to Maine Legislature". *SPPI*. March 24, 2010. *http://www.mast-victims.org/index.php?content=news&action=view&type=newsitem&id=4648*
10. EWG's Guide to Safer Cell Phone Use. "Skip the Radiation Shield." *http://www.ewg.org/cellphoneradiation/8-Safety-Tips*
11. Mae-Wan Ho. "Mobile Phones and Cancer." *Institute of Science in Society*: ISIS. *http://www.i-sis.org.uk/FOI2.php*
12. Press Trust of India. "Can Mobiles cause depression? Cellphone smog could aid depression: Study." *Hindustan Times*, December 15 2005. *http://omega.twoday.net/stories/1267963/* http://www.hindustantimes.com/news/181_1571289,0050.htm
13. "Mobile Phones: an emerging pubic health concern." *Epoch Times*, April 19, 2010. *http://inthesenewtimes.com/2010/04/19/mobile-phones-an-emerging-public-health-concern/*
14. Mortazavi SM et al. Mercury release from dental amalgam restorations after magnetic resonance imaging and following mobile phone use. *Pak J Biol Sci*. 2008 Apr 15;11(8):1142–6. *http://www.ncbi.nlm.nih.gov/pubmed/18819554*
15. Vini Khurana's Web site: Brain-Surgery.us. *http://www.brain-surgery.us/mobilephone.html*
16. Larry Gust. "Wireless phones and Your Health". Gustenviro.com. *http://www.gustenviro.com/cell_phones.html*
17. Sage and Associates. "What to tell your employer about cell phones and PDA's in the workplace—Neurological Effects of Wireless Technologies. Talking Points on Cell Phones and Health Risks." September 2009. *http://www.emfacts.com/2009/09/1131-what-to-tell-your-employer-about-cell-phones-and-pdas-in-the-workplace/*
18. Andrew Michrowski. "New Problems with Cell Phones." Whole Life Expo 2005, Toronto. *http://www.powerwatch.org.uk/pdfs/20060802_michrowski.pdf*
19. "Cell Phone Radiation Dangers—Witness Statement by Andrew Goldsworthy."April 2010. *http://inthesenewtimes.com/2010/05/20/cell-phone-radiation-dangers-witness-statement-by-andrew-goldsworthy/*
20. Sue Kovach. "The Hidden Dangers of Cell Phone Radiation." *Life Extension Magazine*: Report, August 2007. *http://www.lef.org/magazine/mag2007/aug2007_report_cellphone_radiation_02.htm*
21. George Carlo. "Illusion and Escape: The Cell Phone Disease Quagmire. A Summary of American Legal Actions Regarding Mobile Phones and Health Effects." *The American Trial Lawyer*. Fall 2008. *http://www.naturalscience.org/fileadmin/portabledocuments/fact_sheet_no_01.pdf*
22. Neil Cherry. "Cell phone radiation poses a serious biological and health risk." May 7, 2001. *http://ebookbrowse.com/cell-phone-radiation-poses-a-serious-biological-and-health-risk-pdf-d225461507*
23. "Secondhand Cell Phone Radiation," with Cindy Sage. *Your Own Health and Fitness*. Radio Show with Jeffry Fawcett and Layna Berman. Interview: (10.28.2008). *http://www.yourownhealthandfitness.org/?page_id=753*
24. "Mobile Phones and Health: waves and research." *RTD Info: Magazine on European Research*. Issue 46, August 2005. *http://ec.europa.eu/research/rtdinfo/pdf/rtd46_en.pdf*
25. Cindy Sage. "Cell phones and blood brain barrier." CHE-EMF Working Group. EMFacts Consultancy weblog #979. *http://www.emfacts.com/2008/11/979-cell-phones-and-blood-brain-barrier-new-study/*

26. Arthur Firstenberg. "Cell Phones and Wireless Dangers —The fundamentals." October 7, 2007. *http://educate-yourself.org/cn/wirelessandcellphonedangers05oct07.shtml*
27. Olle Johansson. "Today's Research is the reality of tomorrow." April 10, 2006. *http:// www.vws.org/documents/Cell-Project-Documents/2DrJohanssonTodaysResearch_000. pdf*
28. "Summary of a Public Hearing held in Jersey, Channel Islands, UK. February 26, 2007. Expert Witness: Dr George Carlo." *http://www.vws.org/documents/Cell-Project-Documents/9SummaryChannelIslands_000.pdf*
29. Julie A Evans. "The Cell Tolls for Thee: The truth about the cell-phone-cancer link, and what it means for you and your kids." *Best Life*, August 2008. *http://www.giadownloads. com/pdf/MSN_Health_Fitness.pdf*
30. Geoffrey Lean. "Electronic Smog is disrupting nature on a massive scale." *The Independent,* September 7, 2008. *http://www.independent.co.uk/environment/nature/ electronic-smog-is-disrupting-nature-on-a-massive-scale-921711.html?afid=af*
31. Whittow W G et al. Metal objects increase phone radiation: Indicative SAR levels due to an active mobile phone in a front trouser pocket in proximity to common metallic objects. 2008 Loughborough Antennas and Propagation Conference, Loughborough, UK, 17–18 March, pp. 149–152. *https://dspace.lboro.ac.uk/dspace-jspui/handle/2134/3340*
32. "10 Medical Rules Relating to Cellular Telephones." *Omega News*, July 20, 2007. *http:// omega.twoday.net/stories/4089113/*
33. George Carlo, Safe Wireless Initiative. Letter to Eileen O'Connor, EM Radiation Research Trust. October 14, 2006. *http://www.vws.org/documents/Cell-Project-Documen ts/11DrCarlosSafeWirelessinitiative.pdf*
34. "46% of American adults are smartphone owners." Pew Internet: A project of the Pew Research Center. March 1, 2012. *http://www.pewinternet.org/~/media/Files/Reports/2012/Smartphone%20ownership%20 2012.pdf*
35. "Global mobile statistics 2012 Home: all the latest stats on mobile Web, apps, marketing, advertising, subscribers and trends . . ." *mobiThinking*, June 2012. *http://mobithinking. com/mobile-marketing-tools/latest-mobile-stats#subscribers*
36. "How cell phones may cause autism." *Mercola.com*, November 27, 2007. *http://www. next-up.org/pdf/DrMercolaCommentHowCellPhonesMayCauseAutism112007.pdf*
37. Christopher Ketchum. "Warning: Your cell phone may be hazardous to your health." *GQ*, February 2010. *http://www.gq.com/cars-gear/gear-and-gadgets/201002/warning-cell-phone-radiation*
38. Don Maisch. "Mobile Phone Use: It's time to take precautions." *Aust Coll Nut. & Env Med Vol 20* (1) 2001 Apr *http://www.emfacts.com/papers/*
39. Elizabeth Barris. "The Legislator's guide to warning labels on cell phones and the layman's guide to the science behind the non-thermal effects from wireless devices and infrastructure." *The American Association For Cell Phone Safety,* 2011. *http://www. americanassociationforcellphonesafety.org/uploads/Non_Thermal_Paper_10-10_AAA. pdf*
40. "Smartphone Market Hits All-Time Quarterly High Due to Seasonal Strength and Wider Variety of Offerings, According to IDC." Press Release, *International Data Corporation (IDC),* February 6, 2010. *http://www.idc.com/getdoc.jsp?containerId=prUS23299912*
41. "Global mobile statistics 2012 Part A: Mobile subscribers; handset market share; mobile operators." *mobiThinking*, June 2012. *http://mobithinking.com/mobile-marketing-tools/ latest-mobile-stats/a#subscribers*
42. "Global mobile statistics 2012 Part C: Mobile marketing, advertising and messaging." *mobiThinking*, June 2012. *http://mobithinking.com/mobile-marketing-tools/latest-mobile-stats/c*
43. "Global mobile statistics 2012 Part E: Mobile apps, app stores, pricing and failure rates." *mobiThinking,* June 2012. *http://mobithinking.com/mobile-marketing-tools/latest-mobile-stats/e#lotsofapps*
44. "SMS Traffic Break-Out—Regional, 2008-2015." *Portio Research. http://www.scribd. com/doc/55346564/Mobile-Messaging-Futures-2011-2015-Portio-Research-Ltd-EXTRACT-India*
45. "Sleepy connected Americans." *National Sleep Foundation*, March 7, 2011. *http://www. sleepfoundation.org/alert/sleepy-connected-americans*
46. "2009 Sleep in America Poll—Summary of Findings." *National Sleep Foundation, http:// www.sleepfoundation.org/sites/default/files/2009%20Sleep%20in%20America%20 SOF%20EMBARGOED.pdf*

47. "2002 Adult Sleep Habits," *National Sleep Foundation*. *http://www.sleepfoundation.org/article/sleep-america-polls/2002-adult-sleep-habits*
48. Alex Swinkels, National Platform on Radiation Risks. "Italian court ruling on disability from cell/cordless phone use." *EMFacts Consultancy*, December 19, 2009. *http://weepnews.blogspot.com.au/2010/01/disability-court-blames-mobile-phone.html*
49. CNET: Cell phone radiation levels: *www.reviews.cnet.com/cell-phone-radiation-levels*
50. EWG: "Best and Worst Phones" : *www.ewg.org/project/2009cellphone/get-a-safer-phone.php*

Cordless Phones

1. Anne Campbell. "Cordless home phones sparks radiation fear." *Mail Online*, February 6, 2006. *http://www.dailymail.co.uk/health/article-376279/Cordless-home-phones-sparks-radiation-fear.html#ixzz0Q5vvMgEY*
2. "Cordless phones: the unspoken DECT hazard at home and at work." *Tetrawatch*. *http://www.tetrawatch.net/science/dect.php*
3. Haumann T, Sierck P. Non-Stop Pulsed 2.4 GHz Radiation Inside US Homes. 2nd International Workshop on Biological Effects of Electromagnetic Fields 7–11 Oct 2002. *http://2004.uploaded.fresh.co.il/2004/10/13/242805.pdf*
4. Don Maisch. "Medical warnings needed on DECT cordless phone use." *J Aust Coll Nutr & Env Med* 2006 Aug, Vol 25 (2): www.emfacts.com/download/dect.pdf
5. "L Lloyd Morgan on DECT phones." Correspondence with Don Maisch, January 7, 2006. *EMFacts Consultancy*. *http://www.emfacts.com/2006/01/lloyd-morgan-on-dect-phones/*
6. "Request that First Generation DECT Phones be Banned in Canada." Environmental Petition submitted to the Auditor General of Canada, June 2008. Submitted by Magda Havas. *http://www.magdahavas.org/wordpress/wp-content/uploads/2009/10/08_Havas_EPetition_DECT.pdf*
7. Tessa Thomas "After cancer warnings on mobiles, could your home phone be putting your health in Danger?" *Mail Online*, February 18, 2008. *http://www.dailymail.co.uk/health/article-515970/After-cancer-warnings-mobiles-home-phone-putting-health-danger.html*
8. "Digital Cordless Phones: DECT." *Mast Sanity*. http://www.mastsanity.org/index.php?option=com_content&task=view&id=58&Itemid=60
9. Havas M et al. Provocation study using heart rate variability shows microwave radiation from DECT phone affects autonomic nervous system, *Eu J Oncology Library* Vol 5, 273–300. 2010. http://www.avaate.org/article.php3?id_article=2043
10. Alasdair Philips and Jean Philips. "DECT cordless phones (and wi-fi) cause heart irregularities." *Powerwatch*, October 22, 2010. *http://www.powerwatch.org.uk/news/20101022-cordless-heart.asp*
11. "DECT—The Radiation Source at Home: Cordless Phones radiate unnecessarily." German Federal Agency for Radiation Protection Press Release, Jan 31, 2006. *http://getpurepower.ca/Articles/Cell_Towers_Wireless/DECT_Phones/DECT_Radiation_Source_Cordless_Phones.pdf*

Wireless

1. Geoffrey Lean. "Germany warns citizens to avoid using Wi-Fi." *The Independent,* September 9, 2007. *http://www.independent.co.uk/environment/green-living/germany-warns-citizens-to-avoid-using-wifi-401845.html*
2. Gerd Oberfeld "Electromagnetic Pollution in our Environment." Lecture given at the Annual Meeting on behalf of Irish Doctors Environmental Association (IDEA), University of Cork, Ireland, February 2009. *http://www.scribd.com/doc/20828976/Electromagnetic-Pollution-in-Our-Environment*
3. Lynn Quiring. "Wi-Fi and Wi-Max—Why you shouldn't use them." *http://ezinearticles.com/?Wi-fi-and-Wi-max---Why-You-Shouldnt-Use-Them&id=1083187*
4. Olle Johansson. "Wireless Technology and Public Health." Open Letter, *New Era Health and Safety,* May 2009. *http://www.feb.se/ARTICLES/OlleJ.html*
5. Arthur Firstenberg. "The Largest Biological Experiment Ever." *Sun Monthly,* January 1, 2006. *www.mindfully.org/Technology/2006/Firstenberg-EMF-ExperimentJjan06.htm*
6. "Wi-Fi: A Warning Signal." *Panorama,* BBC One, May 21, 2007. *http://news.bbc.co.uk/2/hi/programmes/panorama/6683969.stm*
7. "Wireless Networks (Wi-Fi)." *EMFacts Consultancy* Consumer Health and Safety Advice, Leaflet. *http://www.icems.eu/docs/EMFacts-WIFI.pdf*
8. "DECT cordless phones and Wi-Fi networks." Dirty Electricity. *http://www.dirtyelectricity.ca/dect_phones.htm*
9. Gary Brown. "Wireless Devices, Standards, and Microwave Radiation in the Education Environment." October 2000. *http://www.getpurepower.ca/resources/WireleassDevices_GaryBrown.pdf*
10. Chellis Glendinning. "Trojans! Do Not Trust the Horse. Wireless Mind, Gullible Mind." *Counter Punch,* October 10–12, 2008. *http://www.counterpunch.org/glendinning10122008.html*
11. Andrew Michrowski. "Electromagnetic fields: Questions and answers about wireless technologies." Whole Life Expo 2007, Toronto. November 25, 2007. *http://www.weepinitiative.org/LINKEDDOCS/health/wholelife_emf_2007-0308.pdf*
12. Amy Worthington. "The Radiation Poisoning of America." *Idaho Observer,* October 7, 2007. *http://www.globalresearch.ca/index.php?context=va&aid=7025*
13. Paul Raymond Doyon. "Are the microwaves killing the insects, frogs and birds? And are we next?" *National Health Federation,* February 18, 2008. *http://www.thenhf.com/article.php?id=480*
14. "Wireless Risks in the Mainstream," with Christopher Ketcham and Michael Segell. *Your Own Health and Fitness* Radio Show with Jeffry Fawcett and Layna Berman. Interview: (2.9.2010). *http://www.yourownhealthandfitness.org/?page_id=753*
"Wireless Technology Health News," with Cindy Sage. *Your Own Health and Fitness* Radio Show with Jeffry Fawcett and Layna Berman (10.27.2009). *http://www.yourownhealthandfitness.org/?page_id=753*
"Health Considerations for the Digital Revolution," with B Blake Levitt. *Your Own Health and Fitness* Radio Show with Jeffry Fawcett and Layna Berman (4.24.2012). *http://www.yourownhealthandfitness.org/?page_id=753*
"Wireless Technology Health News," with Cindy Sage. *Your Own Health and Fitness* Radio Show with Jeffry Fawcett and Layna Berman (10.27.2009). *http://www.yourownhealthandfitness.org/?page_id=753*
15. "Alternatives to Wireless Broadband," with Doug Loranger and Sally Hampton. *Your Own Health and Fitness* Radio Show with Jeffry Fawcett and Layna Berman *http://www.yourownhealthandfitness.org/?page_id=753*
16. "Wireless Public Health Crisis," with B Blake Levitt, Jan Newton, and Doug Loranger. *Your Own Health and Fitness* Radio Show with Jeffry Fawcett and Layna Berman (2.7.2006). *http://www.yourownhealthandfitness.org/?page_id=753*
17. "Ill-health from Wi-Fi." Information Sheet 11. *ElectroSensitivity* UK. *http://www.es-uk.info/docs/front-01-ill-health-wifi.pdf*

Wi-MAX and Citywide Wi-Fi

1. Cliff Edwards "Intel's WiMax: Like Wi-Fi on Steroids," *Business Week*, 2005, April 25. *http://www.businessweek.com/magazine/content/05_17/b3930072_mz011.htm*
2. Marsha Walton. "Is 'Wi-Fi' on steroids' really the next big thing?" *CNN.com*, 2006, March 31. *http://edition.cnn.com/2005/TECH/10/17/wireless.wimax/index.html*
3. Deepak Pareek. Wimax: Taking Wireless to the Max. (Auerbach Publications, 2006)
4. Gemma Simpson. "Manchester plans UK's biggest citywide Wi-Fi network." *ZDNet Asia*, December 1, 2006. *http://www.zdnet.com/manchester-plans-uks-biggest-citywide-wi-fi-network-3040149717/*
5. "Clearwire Launches WiMAX Network in Las Vegas." *Cellular-news*, July 21, 2009. *http://www.cellular-news.com/story/38669.php*
6. "Clearwire Launches WiMAX Network in Atlanta City." *Cellular-news*, 2009. June 16. *http://www.cellular-news.com/story/38024.php*
7. Tim Conneally. "Clearwire subscribers to get WiMAX coverage in Moscow and Tokyo." September 14, 2009. *Betanews.com*. *http://www.betanews.com/article/Clearwire-subscribers-to-get-WiMAX-coverage-in-Moscow-Tokyo/1252967950*
8. Marguerite Reardon. "Spring to launch WiMax service in September." *CNET News*, 2008, June 18. *http://news.cnet.com/8301-10784_3-9972229-7.html*
9. Rakesh Kumar Jha. "WiMAX and Beyond WiMAX Technology." *Ezinearticles.com*. *http://ezinearticles.com/?WiMAX-and-Beyond-WiMAX-Technology&id=4280744*
10. Richard Latker. "Exposure to invisible cloud of energy called electrosmog is rising." *New York Times*, 2007, September 24. *http://www.nytimes.com/2007/09/23/business/worldbusiness/23iht-wirelessbox.4.7611175.html*
11. Lynn Quiring. "Wi-Fi and Wi-Max—Why you shouldn't use them." *Ezinearticles. com*. *http://ezinearticles.com/?Wi-fi-and-Wi-max---Why-You-Shouldnt-Use-Them&id=1083187*
12. "Wi-Max, the Next Wireless Exposure," with Libby Kelley. Your Own Health and Fitness Radio Show with Jeffry Fawcett and Layna Berman. (12.4.2007). *http://www.yourownhealthandfitness.org/?page_id=753*

Children

1. Alasdair Philips and Jean Philips. "Young children's use of mobile phones soars in the UK." *Powerwatch*. January 11, 2010. *http://www.powerwatch.org.uk/news/20100111_mobile_phones_kids.asp*
2. "Dr George Carlo on Children and Health Damage from Mobile Phones." *Mast Sanity* *http://www.mastsanity.org/home/2/280-dr-george-carlo-on-children-and-health-damage-from-mobile-phones.html*
3. "Is Wi-Fi safe for children? Dr George Carlo speaks on Wi-Fi Radiation in Schools." *safeinschool.org*, 2011 March 24. *http://www.safeinschool.org/2011/03/dr.html*
4. Don Maisch. "Children and Mobile Phones . . . Is There a Health Risk? " *Aust Coll Nut. & Env Med* 2001 Aug Vol 22 (2) 3–8. *www.emfacts.com/download/children_mobiles.pdf*
5. "Children and Mobile Phones: The Health of The Following Generations Is in Danger." Decision of Russian National Committee of Non-Ionizing Radiation Protection: 2008 Report, April 14, 2008, Page 3. *http://www.who.int/peh-emf/project/mapnatreps/RUSSIA%20report%202008.pdf*
6. Independent Expert Group on Mobile Phones. "Mobile Phones and Health: Chairman Sir William Stewart" ("The Stewart Report") 2000 April. Report: *http://www.teiser.gr/icd_old/sar/iegmp.pdf*
   Summary and Recommendations: *http://www.iegmp.org.uk/documents/iegmp_1.pdf*
7. "Kids mobile phone ads 'Irresponsible' *BBC News*, 2001, September 4. *http://news.bbc.co.uk/2/hi/in_depth/sci_tech/2001/glasgow_2001/1525676.stm*
8. "German Academy of Pediatrics: Keep Kids Away from Mobiles," *Microwave News*, Vol 21 (4) 5, Jan/Feb 2001. *http://microwavenews.com/news/backissues/j-f01issue.pdf*
9. R C Kane. A Possible Association Between Fetal/neonatal Exposure to Radiofrequency Electromagnetic Radiation and the Increased Incidence of Autism Spectrum Disorders (ASD). *Med Hypotheses*. 2004;62(2):195–7. *http://www.ncbi.nlm.nih.gov/pubmed/14962625*

10. "What Cell Phones Can Do to a Youngster's Brain in 2 Minutes. The Child Scrambler." *Sunday Mirror,* April 1, 2004. *http://www.scribd.com/doc/3121224/What-Cell-Phones-Can-Do-To-A-Youngsters-Brain-In-2-Minutes*
11. "Children and cell phones: Time to start talking sense," *Microwave News,* 2010 May 3. *http://microwavenews.com/news-center/children-and-cell-phones-time-start-talking-sense*
12. "Thai Minister mulls cellphone ban for youngsters," *Channel News Asia,* 2002 April 5. http://www.mastaction.co.uk/news/Thai-minister-mulls-cellphone-ban-for-youngsters/
13. "Bangladesh to ban mobile phones for Children, Industry Outraged." *Associated Press* 2002 June 3, *http://www.goaegis.com/articles/associated_press_060302_w6q2m9g3b.html*
14. Alasdair Philips and Jean Philips. "Children and Mobile Phones 1: Use of mobile phones by young people." Powerwatch. *http://www.powerwatch.org.uk/library/downloads/children-phones-1-use-2012-03.pdf*
15. Alasdair Philips and Jean Philips. "Children and Mobile Phones 2: Official Advice across the world." *Powerwatch.* March 2012. *http://www.powerwatch.org.uk/library/downloads/children-phones-2-advice-2012-03.pdf*
16. Alasdair Philips and Jean Philips. "Children and Mobile Phones 3: The Research". *Powerwatch. http://www.powerwatch.org.uk/library/downloads/children-phones-3-research-2012-03.pdf*
17. "German Academy of Pediatrics: Keep Kids Away from Mobiles," *Microwave News,* Vol 21 (4) 5, Jan/Feb 2001.
18. "Important New Russian Research on Cell Phone Radiation's Effect on Cognitive and Other Functions in Children." *Electromagnetic Health* 04.11.2011. *http://electromagnetichealth.org/electromagnetic-health-blog/russian-res-children-emf/*
19. Generation M2. Media in the Lives of 8- to 18-year-olds. *A Kaiser Family Foundation Study.* January 2010. *http://www.kff.org/entmedia/upload/8010.pdf*
20. Centers for Disease Control and Prevention. Prevalence of Autism Spectrum Disorders—Autism and Developmental Disabilities Monitoring Network, 14 Sites, United States, 2008. *Surveillance Summaries.* March 30, 2012 / 61(SS03);1-19. *http://www.cdc.gov/ncbddd/autism/data.html*
21. BioInitiative Working Group, Cindy Sage and David O Carpenter, Editors. BioInitiative 2012: Biologically-based Exposure Standards for Low-Intensity Electromagnetic Radiation at www.bioinitiative.org <*http://www.bioinitiative.org*>, December 31, 2012. Summary for the Public (2012 Supplement)

Wireless in Schools

1. Gary Brown. "Wireless Devices, Standards, and Microwave Radiation in the Education Environment," October 2000. *http://www.getpurepower.ca/resources/WireleassDevices_GaryBrown.pdf*
2. "Safe Schools 2012: Medical and Scientific Experts Call For Safe Technologies in Schools." A document for schools. *Wifiinschools.org.uk http://wifiinschools.org.uk/resources/safeschools2012.pdf*
3. "Wireless technologies and young people: A resource for schools." *Wifiinschools.org.uk* October 2011. *http://wifiinschools.org.uk/resources/wireless+technologies+and+young+people+Oct2011.pdf*
4. Russell Campbell. "Wi-Fi in schools: a threat to your child's health?" *ni4kidsd.com,* November 2008. *http://www.ni4kids.com/features/article.aspx?listing_id=d5bdd25f-90bc-41c1-aeb1-f974ab325edf&cat_id=6f4911ae-9396-4932-94b4-f541b4215a20*
5. "Key points for schools." *Wifiinschools.org.uk. www.wifiinschools.org.uk/9.html*
6. "Dr Andrew Goldsworthy on Wi-Fi in Schools." *EMFacts Consultancy,* November 9, 2011. *http://www.emfacts.com/2011/11/dr-andrew-goldsworthy-on-wi-fi-in-schools/*
7. "Schools guide: Wi-fi in Schools." *Wired Child. http://wiredchild.org/schools.html*

8. Michael Bevington of Stowe School. "Wi-Fi in the Classroom: Health Advice to schools" *http://www.scribd.com/doc/24004604/Wi-Fi-in-the-Classroom-Health-Advice-to-Schools*

9. Lyndsay Young. "Parents threaten to remove children from Formby school over wi-fi installation." *Liverpoool Daily Post*, 21 October 2009. *http://www.liverpooldailypost.co.uk/liverpool-news/regional-news/2009/10/21/parents-threaten-to-remove-children-from-formby-school-over-wi-fi-installation-92534-24979296/*

10. Alasdair Philips and Jean Philips. "Wireless Technology in Schools." *http://www.powerwatch.org.uk/library/downloads/schools-wireless-20111018.pdf*

11. Nic Fleming. "Warning on Wi-Fi health risk to Children." *The Telegraph*, April 28, 2007. *http://www.telegraph.co.uk/news/uknews/1549944/Warning-on-wi-fi-health-risk-to-children.html*

12. Nic Fleming. "Wi-Fi risks in schools must be reviewed." *Daily Telegraph*, 21 May 2007. *http://www.telegraph.co.uk/news/uknews/1552205/Wi-Fi-risks-in-schools-must-be-reviewed.html*

13. "Suspend wi-fi in schools says union chief following reports it causes ill-health." *Daily Mail*, 28 July 2008. *http://www.dailymail.co.uk/news/article-1039235/Suspend-wi-fi-schools-says-union-chief-following-reports-causes-ill-health.html*

14. "Dr George Carlo speaks on Wi-Fi Radiation in Schools." *safeinschool.org*. March 24, 2011. *http://www.safeinschool.org/2011/03/dr.html*

15. "Wi-fi worry." *BBC News*, December 13, 2006. *http://news.bbc.co.uk/2/hi/uk_news/magazine/6172257.stm*

16. Alec Liu. *"Experts: Wi-Worry About Wi-Fi Danger?" Fox News, August 18, 2010. http://www.foxnews.com/scitech/2010/08/18/wi-fi-making-sick/*

17. Magda Havas. "Open Letter to Parents, Teachers, School Boards. Regarding Wi-Fi Networks in Schools." May 2, 2012. *http://www.magdahavas.com/wordpress/wp-content/uploads/2012/05/Wi-Fi-Open-Letter2012.pdf*

18. Magda Havas. "Open Letter to Medical Officer of Health—Wi-Fi in schools." September 29, 2010. *http://www.magdahavas.com/open-letter-to-medical-officer-of-health-about-wifi-in-schools/*

19. Gerd Oberfeld. "WLAN and DECT in schools and kindergartens." Open letter, December 5, 2005. *http://www.dirtyelectricity.ca/images/Salzburg%20bans%20wi-fi%20and%20DECT.pdf*

20. "WiFi in Schools a Health Hazard." Olle Johansson's letter to the Greater Victoria School District—Committee on Wi-Fi, February 11, 2011. *http://www.heartmdinstitute.com/wireless-safety/why-get-wired-schools*

21. "2012 Expert Witness Testimonies to U.S. Court concerning Removal of Wi-Fi in Public Schools." *safeinschool.org*. April 28, 2012. *http://www.safeinschool.org/2012/04/updated-2012-expert-witness-testimonies.html*

22. Geoffrey Lean. "Wi-Fi backlash. Councils urge caution on networks in schools." *The Independent,* July 16, 2007. *http://nomoremasts.blogspot.com.au/2007/07/wi-fi-backlash-councils-urge-caution-on.html*

23. BioInitiative Working Group, Cindy Sage and David O Carpenter, Editors. BioInitiative 2012: Biologically-based Exposure Standards for Low-Intensity Electromagnetic Radiation at www.bioinitiative.org *<http://www.bioinitiative.org>*, December 31, 2012. Conclusions.

24. Working for Safe Technologies for Nurseries, Schools and Colleges. *Wi-Fi in schools:. www.wifiinschools.org.uk*

Research Headlines

1. George Carlo, Head of CTIA Research Project: Presentation of Findings in 1999. "Cellphones and Brain Tumors: 15 Reasons for Concern, Science, Spin and the Truth Behind Interphone. Quotations from Scientists, Physicians and others." L Lloyd Morgan, primary author. International EMF Collaborative. August 25, 2009, 7. *http://archive.radiationresearch.org/pdfs/reasons_quotes.pdf*. *http://www.radiationresearch.org/pdfs/reasons_us.pdf*

2. Khurana et al. Cell phones and brain tumors: A review including the long-term epidemiologic data. *Surg Neurol.* 2009 Sep;72(3):205–14.
3. "Cellphones and Brain Tumors: 15 Reasons for Concern, Science, Spin and the Truth Behind Interphone. Quotations from Scientists, Physicians and others." L Lloyd Morgan, primary author. International EMF Collaborative. August 25, 2009, 9. *http://archive. radiationresearch.org/pdfs/reasons_quotes.pdf. http://www.radiationresearch.org/pdfs/ reasons_us.pdf*
4. Burch et al. Melatonin metabolite excretion among cellular telephone users. *Int J Radiat Biol.* 2002 Nov;78(11):1029–36.
5. Vecchio F et al. Mobile phone emission modulates inter-hemispheric functional coupling of EEG alpha rhythms in elderly compared to young subjects. *Clin Neurophysiol.* 2010 Feb;121(2):163–71.
6. Cindy Sage. Are Bluetooth devices really safer than using a cell phone? EMFacts *Consultancy. http://www.emfacts.com/2012/08/are-bluetooth-devices-really-safer-than- using-a-cell-phone/*
7. Gursatej Gandhi A. Genetic damage in mobile phone users: some preliminary findings. *Indian Journal of Human Genetics,* 2005, Vol: 11, 2 : 99–104.
8. Mortazavi SM et al. Mercury release from dental amalgam restorations after magnetic resonance imaging and following mobile phone use. *Pak J Biol Sci.* 2008 Apr 15;11(8):1142–6.
9. Lai et al. Naltrexone blocks RFR-induced DNA double strand breaks in rat brain cells. *Wireless Networks,* 1997 Dec; Vol 3 (6) 471–476.
10. Huber R et al. Exposure to pulse-modulated radio frequency electromagnetic fields affects regional cerebral blood flow. *Eur J Neurosci.* 2005 Feb;21(4):1000–6.
11. Arnetz BB et al. Effects from 884 MHz mobile phone radiofrequency on brain electrophysiology, sleep, cognition, and well-being. Conference proceedings. *http:// microwavenews.com/october-29-2007*
12. Hallberg O, Johansson O. Alzheimer Mortality—why does it increase so fast in sparsely populated areas? *European Biology and Bioelectromagnetics.* 2005; 1: 225–246.
13. Schüz J et al. Risks for central nervous system diseases among mobile phone subscribers: a Danish retrospective cohort study. *PLoS One.* 2009;4(2):e4389.
14. Divan HA et al. Prenatal and postnatal exposure to cell phone use and behavioral problems in children. *Epidemiology.* 2008 May 7.
15. Rezk AY et al. Fetal and neonatal responses following maternal exposure to mobile phones. *Saudi Med J.* 2008 Feb;29(2):218–23.
16. Klieeisen M. What A Cell Phone Can Do To A Child's Brain In Just Two Minutes. Spanish Neuro Diagnostic Research Institute in Marbella. *http://www.rense.com/ general18/cell.htm*
17. Abramson MJ et al. Mobile telephone use is associated with changes in cognitive function in young adolescents. *Bioelectromagnetics.* 2009 Dec;30(8):678–86.
18. Several Studies on the effect of radiation on children's brains:
    a. Gandhi O et al. Electromagnetic Absorption in the Human Head and Neck for Mobile Telephones at 835 and 1900 MHz. *IEEE transactions on microwave theory and techniques,* 1996 Oct, Vol 44 (10).
    b. Christ A et al. Age-dependent tissue-specific exposure of cell phone users. *Phys Med Biol.* 2010 Apr 7;55(7):1767–83.
    c. Christ A et al. Impact of pinna compression on the RF absorption in the heads of adult and juvenile cell phone users. *Bioelectromagnetics.* 2010 Mar 30.
    d. Wiart J et al. Analysis of RF exposure in the head tissues of children and adults. *Phys. Med. Biol.* 53 3681.
    e. Fernandez C.R et al. Comparison of electromagnetic absorption characteristics in the head of adult and a children for 1800 MHz mobile phones. *IEEE MTT-S* International Conference 2004.
    f. Martínez-Búrdalo M et al. Comparison of FDTD-calculated specific absorption rate in adults and children when using a mobile phone at 900 and 1800 MHz. *Phys Med Biol.* 2004 Jan 21;49(2):345–54.

19. Erogul O et al. Effects of electromagnetic radiation from a cellular phone on human sperm motility: an in vitro study. *Arch Med Res*. 2006 Oct;37(7):840–3. *http://drwdowin. com/CellPhonesAndSpermMotility.pdf*
20. De Iuliis GN et al. Mobile phone radiation induces reactive oxygen species production and DNA damage in human spermatozoa in vitro. *PLoS One*. 2009 Jul 31;4(7):e6446.
21. Eger H et al, 2004. The Influence of Being Physically Near to a Cell Phone Transmission Mast on the Incidence of Cancer. *Umwelt Medizin Gesellschaft* 17,4 2004.
22. Santini R et al. Study on the health of people living near mobile telephone relay stations: I/Incidence according to distance and sex. *Pathol Biol (Paris)*. 2002 Jul;50(6):369–73.
23. Cindy Sage. BioInitiative Report, August 2007. Section 1: Public Summary for the Public, 13. *http://www.bioinitiative.org/freeaccess/report/docs/section_1.pdf*
24. BioInitiative Working Group, Cindy Sage and David O. Carpenter, Editors. BioInitiative 2012: Biologically-based Exposure Standards for Low-Intensity Electromagnetic Radiation at www.bioinitiative.org December 31, 2012. Summary for the Public (2012 Supplement)

All references and links correct at the time of writing.

About the Author

Due to a long period of illness, Alison started to learn as much as she could about the ways in which *how* we live affects our health. As the mother of a young boy who also became ill due to environmental causes, she decided to help spread the word about the fact that it's not only how we live that can determine our health, but also *where* we live.

Waving goodbye to her former life in marketing and manufacturing, she trained as a Building Biology professional in the US. She has combined their knowledge with her own research, consulting, qualifications, and in-field experience, and married this with the very latest news from science and technology. And along the way, she managed to recover not only her son's health but also her own.

Since the end of the last century (!) Alison has spent years travelling extensively (both on the Internet and inside a plane) to learn from the leaders in many related fields. This has resulted in a unique way of working, and a deep understanding of how we can change our environments to optimise our health and vitality.

Alison was born in the UK and started her working life in London. She and her husband have called Australia home since the 80's, and are now lucky enough to live on the edge of the Pacific Ocean in Sydney

I'D JUST LIKE TO SAY A BIG "THANK YOU!" TO:

Everyone who encouraged and sustained me along the long road of producing this book. Of particular importance were:

Vicki Warren who shared her very limited time to talk and listen and answer and expand and read and comment. . . It's made all the difference in the world. This really wouldn't be here without her help.

George Carlo has consistently made space in his extremely busy schedule to answer questions and give incisive, constructive, encouraging and supportive feedback. To say it's been much appreciated is a huge understatement.

Everyone at the **Institute of Building Biology** in the US who helped to play a part in my learning about this incredible subject: from **Larry Gust**, **Spark Burmaster,** and **Martine Davis** at that very first IBE course, to all the other building biologists who so generously shared their time and knowledge, and continue to show others how to turn their homes into healthy havens. (A special thanks to Larry for persuading me to take that first trip over to the US, and then continuing to be so helpful.)

Robyn Walker and **Joelle Shelhot,** whose help has been beyond uplifting. And inspiring. And motivating. Their consistent encouragement has helped me keep going when this incredibly long project has hit patches where it's all seemed just a little bit too overwhelming. I'd like to thank them both for everything they've done to help smooth over the bits that were bumpy, and in sharing the celebrations when things flowed smoothly.

Pam Booth, Robyn Rowlison and **Michelle McCallum,** for all their reading and feedback and support - and of course, friendship.

John Lincoln of EMR Surveys in Sydney, for sharing endless cups of coffee up at the Heights, and taking time out to have a natter about work and the world.

My parents, **Pat and Vernon**, for their care and generosity, and for giving me such a valuable foundation in life.

Oliver and **Toby,** for listening and taking notice, keeping things grounded and real, and continuing to be my greatest teachers (always in the kindest and most gentle ways possible!).

Elena and **Lucy,** for their care, interest and help (and for generally being extremely good news to have around.)

And most importantly to **Tim**, for his unending kindness, support, and encouragement to step up to the plate. He continues to redefine strength, generosity, and patience.

I also want to thank *you* - for choosing this book. Please help to make a difference by sharing all that you learn with those that you love - and perhaps even those that you don't!

Don't forget the Companion Book

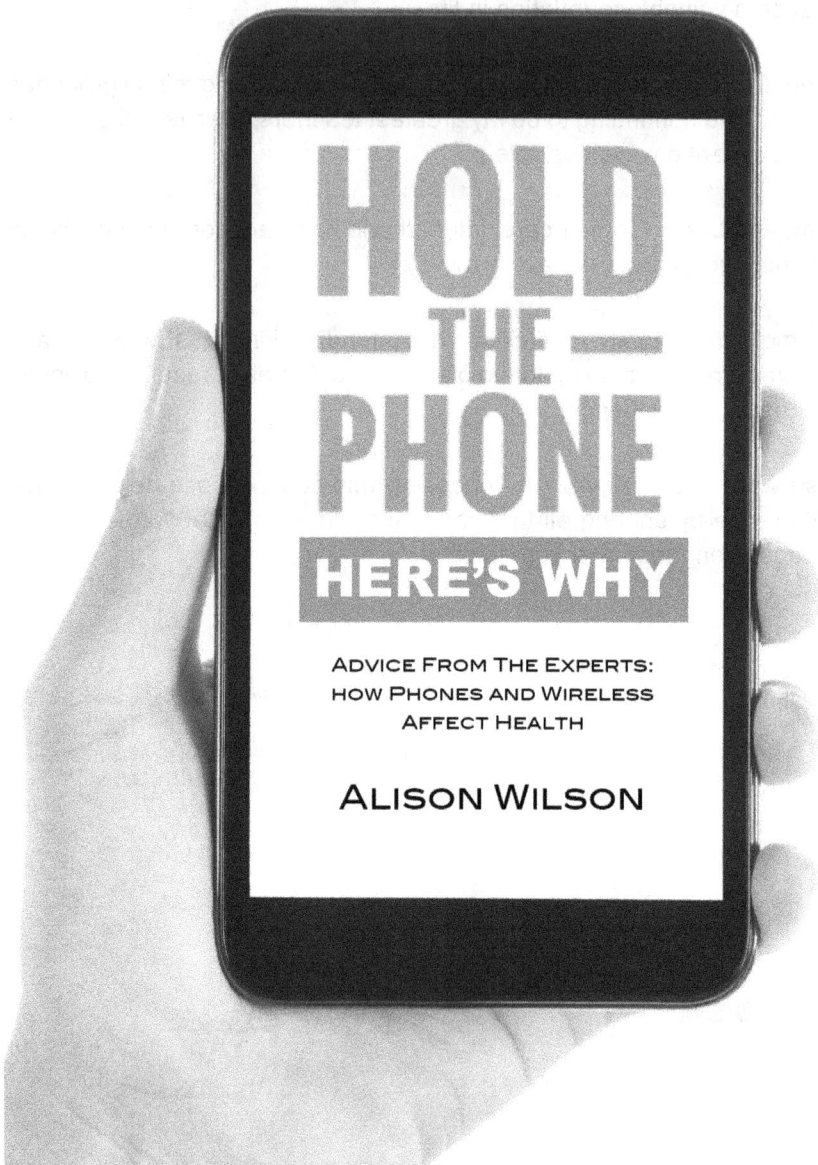

HOLD
— THE —
PHONE

HERE'S WHY

ADVICE FROM THE EXPERTS:
HOW PHONES AND WIRELESS
AFFECT HEALTH

ALISON WILSON

Hold the Phone: Here's Why

This is the other half of the story: the important information about how phones and wireless affect health.

Based on advice from the leading experts and scientists "*Hold The Phone: Here's Why*" is an essential guidebook that shows you *why* it's so important to protect your health from the radiation emitted by mobile phones, cordless phones and all things 'wireless'. It will tell you:

> ➤ *What the concerns are about using phones and 'wireless';*
> ➤ *how they affect your health*
> ➤ *what the early warning symptoms look like;*
> ➤ *all about 'electrosensitivity', and just how many it's affecting*
> ➤ *how much research is available,*
> ➤ *what the studies have found;*
> ➤ *which governments have issued official warnings;*
> ➤ *who are the reliable sources you can trust for accurate information;*

"Knowledge is power" has particular relevance here. And this is precisely why this knowledge-conveyance book by Alison Wilson should be read by, and remain on the bookshelf of, every parent, spouse, and friend of every person who uses mobile communication devices. Alison has done what governments, scientists and industry have so far failed to do: empower consumers to make their own informed safety choices about wireless communication devices."

George L Carlo

" A great summary of the state of the science. More than that, it is an excellent reference document. I think that for parents this is a must-read book for protecting their children's health in the growing wireless environment."

Don Maisch *(EMFacts Consultancy)*

INDEX

More information, and updates, can be found at

www.holdthephone.co

"I am a firm believer in the people.

*If given the truth, they can be depended upon
to meet any national crisis.*

The great point is to bring them the real facts."

Abraham Lincoln